They Can't Find Anything Wrong!

THEY CAN'T FIND ANYTHING WRONG!

7 Keys to Understanding, Treating, and Healing Stress Illness

David D. Clarke, M.D.

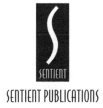

SENTIENT PUBLICATIONS

Cover design by Kim Johansen, Black Dog Design
Book design by Timm Bryson and Alfred Hicks

Library of Congress Cataloging-in-Publication Data

Clarke, David D., 1953-
They can't find anything wrong! : 7 keys to understanding, treating & healing stress illness / by David D. Clarke.
    p. cm.
ISBN 978-1-59181-064-3
1. Stress (Psychology) 2. Stress (Psychology)—Health aspects. 3. Stress management. 4. Medicine, Psychosomatic. I. Title.

    RC455.4.S87C553 2007
    616.9'8—dc22
        2007013430

Printed in the United States of America

10 9 8 7 6 5 4 3 2 1

SENTIENT PUBLICATIONS
A Limited Liability Company
1113 Spruce Street
Boulder, CO 80302
www.sentientpublications.com

*It is more important to know what sort of person
has a disease, than what sort of disease a person has.*

—Hippocrates (460 – 377 BCE)

CONTENTS

ACKNOWLEDGEMENTS

Many people provided generous support to the writing of this book. My immediate and extended family listened for countless hours and provided helpful comments. My patients answered the most personal questions and shared difficult moments of their lives.

Christine Kris showed me how to find the meaning in the smallest personal details.

David Fainer taught me that before ordering a medical test, I should always know what I would do for the patient if the test was normal or abnormal. He pointed out that if the answer was the same either way, then the test was unnecessary.

William Snape knows that stress causes real symptoms and that effective treatment is possible. Few physicians understand this as well as he does.

Harriet Kaplan was unsurpassed at finding and relieving the stresses that cause illness.

Ian MacMillan and Charles Zerzan know that the care of stress illness patients takes time and provided support at key moments in my evolution as a physician.

Barry Cadish and Sarah Willett devoted time and hard work to the manuscript far beyond the call of friendship.

The personal warmth, knowledge, experience, energy and professionalism of Mim Eichler-Rivas influenced every chapter.

My professional colleagues provide the finest medical care that I know. It has been a privilege to work with and learn from them. It is difficult to imagine another group of clinicians and nurses who could have supported my work with stress illness patients as well.

Lynn Hanson suggested some of the references in the appendix and Marlene Smith found the Hippocrates quotation that opens the book.

I owe a great debt to the people who reviewed the manuscript and provided thoughtful, detailed suggestions: Shirley Barker, Eileen Brady, Melanie Camras, Jack G. Clarke, Lucas M. Clarke, Vincent J. Felitti, Peter Fish, Linda Hedge, April Henry, Susan Hook, Marcia Liberson, Sharon Maxey, Linda Moraga, Sonya Richards, Herb Salomon, Stephen Stolzberg and Nancy Ward.

AUTHOR'S NOTE

To honor the privacy and confidentiality of my patients, in telling their stories I changed their names, the names of family and friends and all personal details that could identify them. At times, I combined the experiences of two or more similar patients into a single story. All passages have been reviewed by the patients where possible prior to publication.

If you have symptoms, including but not limited to any that resemble symptoms described in this book, you should visit your doctor for a full evaluation. This book may be useful in discussing potential causative factors with your doctor but should not be used in lieu of medical advice from a health care professional. The reader agrees to hold the author and any agents, partner's agents, licensees and assigns harmless from any liability, claim, cost, damage or expense (including reasonable attorney's fees) arising out of or in connection with the sale, transfer or use of this book.

PART I
A NEW LOOK AT AN INVISIBLE ILLNESS

The real act of discovery consists not in finding new lands, but in seeing with new eyes.

—Marcel Proust

CHAPTER 1
WHAT IS YOUR BODY TRYING TO TELL YOU?

It's not what you're eating; it's what's eating you.

—Janet Greeson

A BAFFLING ILLNESS

ELLEN HAD LOST ALL HOPE. MARRIED, IN HER LATE FORTIES, A MOTHER OF TWO teenage daughters, and a director of a major metropolitan library system, Ellen introduced herself by looking up from her hospital bed and saying wearily, "Don't waste your time with me, Doctor. They've been trying to diagnose me for fifteen years and my tests are always normal." She went on to describe the pattern that her attacks followed, promising that this episode would be over in a few days. Then Ellen sighed and spoke words I have heard countless times in my practice: "They can't find anything wrong!" Evaluations by over a dozen specialists and sixty separate hospital stays at a prestigious university medical center had failed to uncover the cause of her debilitating symptoms or give her any relief. Fortunately, and much to Ellen's surprise, a little over an hour later I was able to cure her illness.

You or someone you know could be suffering from a similarly baffling disease. Every year in the United States, health care providers receive hundreds of millions of visits from adults seeking causes and cures for a range of ailments. Incredibly, up to half of these patients remain undiagnosed and inadequately treated, because tests and examinations "can't find anything wrong," even though the pain and changes in body function are perfectly real. Among the symptoms that patients like Ellen experience are:

- Pain such as headache, back pain, neck pain, chest pain, muscle or joint pain, and abdominal pain
- Abnormal swallowing, digestion, or bowel function including constipation, diarrhea, and bloating
- Nausea or vomiting
- Discomfort in the bladder or during urination
- Respiratory symptoms, including difficulty breathing and cough
- Voice changes
- Heart palpitations
- Pelvic and vaginal irritation, premenstrual or menstrual pain
- Fatigue
- Abnormal sleeping or eating
- Symptoms related to nerve function such as blurred vision, dizziness, ringing in the ears, itching of the skin, sweating, numbness or tingling

These symptoms are the body's way of letting us know something is wrong. Diseases that we diagnose with tests also can cause these symptoms – diseases we can describe as *visible* illnesses – so it is frustrating as well as baffling when x-rays, scans, endoscopes, blood tests, and other studies cannot find the cause. Tragically, millions of patients like Ellen suffer symptoms from an invisible cause for years, even decades, without remedy, resolution, or relief. Now, however, this is changing. We have learned that by asking the right questions, it is possible to find answers and diagnoses, which lead to treatments and cures. After working in this field for more than two decades, with experience in diagnosis and treatment of more than seven thousand patients like Ellen, I can attest to the fact that real hope is on the way.

For Ellen, relief came almost immediately – in the span of one interview – primarily because of her willingness to share details of her life no one had asked about before. At first, she repeated her medical history in a detached, rehearsed way. Every few months for fifteen years, Ellen suffered mysterious attacks of abdominal pain, dizziness, and vomiting lasting for days. These episodes were as unpredictable as they were severe. The attacks could strike at work or when she was watching her daughters play soccer or while preparing a meal for her family. Ellen's life went on hold until the symptoms subsided. Shaking her head, she referred again to the countless examinations, diagnostic tests, and even a psychiatric evaluation that failed to reveal any abnormality. Each time, an attack would end as suddenly as it had begun. Between episodes, Ellen felt completely well.

As I searched for the cause of her condition, our conversation soon moved in directions Ellen had not anticipated. Her demeanor changed as she became increasingly emotional and animated, while her eyes filled with the light of self-discovery. The mystery we unraveled and the principles employed to understand and relieve her invisible illness are the subject of this book. After I identified the source of her problem, she never had another attack.

Stress caused Ellen's symptoms, just as it causes a variety of symptoms in millions of patients today. Physicians use many terms for this condition but I call it, simply, stress illness. Before we look at the specific clues that Ellen provided in telling her story, let us talk further about what stress illness *is* – and *isn't* – and why it is woefully misunderstood by so many health care professionals.

STRESS ILLNESS: A 21ST CENTURY EPIDEMIC

Medical science has long recognized the negative impact of stress on our daily lives. In the 1980s, there was an upsurge in interest about stress as a component of both physical and psychological diseases. Today, it seems like nearly everyone complains about our increasingly stressful 21st century existence. Unfortunately, stress is treated as a lifestyle issue, something we have to learn to manage – like our bank accounts or our busier than ever schedules. Rarely mentioned is the idea that powerful hidden forces might be undermining our best efforts to cope. In addition, the problem of physical symptoms caused by stress never became a significant part of the training of physicians. Only a handful of physicians have taken a closer look at the ways in which stress is literally making millions of people sick.

In stress illness, one or more of five types of stress – prolonged effects from stress in childhood, current stress, post-traumatic stress, depression, and anxiety – causes physical symptoms. Sufferers are often unaware of the nature or degree of the stress that makes them ill. Symptoms can occur anywhere in the body and can be just as severe as symptoms caused by any other disease, but x-rays and blood tests cannot detect the cause. Successful diagnosis and treatment are possible but, unfortunately, when diagnostic tests are normal, many doctors do not know what to look for next. Consequently, stress illness patients often suffer needlessly for years or even decades.

Physicians use a variety of labels for symptoms when they cannot find a cause, but these do not capture the essence of this disease as well as the term I prefer, stress illness. "Functional disorder," for example, refers to the fact that symptoms result from abnormal function of an organ rather than abnormal anatomy, yet this term fails to include the crucial role of stress. The term "psychosomatic disease" describes the interaction of mind (psyche) and body (soma) but it suggests to many patients that their symptoms aren't real, or that somehow personal deficiencies are to blame for their condition, and neither of these is the case. A term used by mental health professionals is "somatoform disorder," which describes illness that resembles or masquerades as a disease of the body but is, at the core, a psychological disorder. Again, the role of stress is not included. Finally and worst of all, stress illness patients can hear, "It's all in your head," as if their symptoms are imaginary.

Regardless of the name given to this condition, it is an unfortunate fact that some physicians believe stress illness is not part of their responsibility to diagnose or treat. One doctor subjected a patient to nine months of diagnostic tests without once asking about stress. After I successfully treated the patient's stress illness the doctor sent me a note that said, "It is reassuring to know I didn't miss anything important." Any one of thousands of patients I have treated for stress illness would gladly explain to this doctor the importance of what she missed. It is surprising that some physicians have this attitude, because stress causes the symptoms in up to half of their patients.

This problem exists because medical school and hospital residency instruction focuses on diseases that doctors can detect with blood tests, scans, endoscopes, biopsies, and other diagnostic tools. When these tests are normal, many doctors are not sure what to do and might order more tests, refer to a specialist, or tell patients they "can't find anything wrong." Other doctors resort to an approach described by Alan Barbour, M.D., the late director of the Stanford University General Medicine Clinic. In his carefully researched book *Caring for Patients*, Dr. Barbour explains that physicians often label stress illness symptoms with meaningless terms that distract attention from the real problem (some examples of these terms are in the next paragraph). These terms are labels and not diagnoses because they fail to suggest any further evaluation, they do not lead to useful treatment, and there is no way to confirm them.

Stress illness, on the other hand, is a diagnosis that demands further investigation to find the stress responsible for the symptoms. And here's where the promising news comes for you and anyone suffering from stress illness. After identification of the stress (or stresses), treatment options are nearly always available. Many (though not all) patients labeled with irritable bowel syndrome, fibromyalgia, temporomandibular joint disorder, functional dyspepsia, spastic dysphonia, idiopathic chest pain, pelvic congestion syndrome, and a long list of other terms find substantial relief after identification and treatment of key stresses in their lives. Relieving symptoms by treating stress is what confirms the diagnosis of stress illness.

I must caution you that Ellen's stress illness was relieved more readily than most. However, the process by which we found her diagnosis and cure is a good beginning for your understanding of stress illness.

READING THE BODY'S MESSAGE: ELLEN'S STORY

Ellen reported that when her symptoms began she was in her early thirties, very happily married, with a degree in library sciences. She was moving up the managerial ladder and in excellent health. Then, out of the blue – as she described it – she developed the illness that was to frustrate her and a major university hospital for fifteen years. The symptoms themselves were straightforward: six to ten times a year she experienced attacks of severe dizziness, vomiting, and abdominal pain that would last from one to four days. Between attacks, she felt fine. Ellen required hospitalization for about half her attacks. Although the symptoms started in adulthood, the cause came much earlier.

As our exchange began, Ellen was skeptical about the value of retelling her story. With an air of hopelessness, she interjected that I shouldn't waste my time, because she was certain I couldn't help. Ellen's husband sat quietly next to her, resigned to hearing an account he had listened to many times. Ellen explained that she was visiting relatives in southern Washington State (near where I practice). In her hometown of Seattle, every physician in the departments of Ear, Nose & Throat; Gastroenterology; and Neurology at the university medical center had seen her, not to mention a psychiatrist who ruled out any mental health problems. Whenever such thorough evaluations find nothing, it is a major clue that the patient could be suffering from stress illness.

As we talked about the frequency and duration of her symptoms, Ellen didn't add much to the description above except for one remarkable fact: "One of the odd things is that I always got an attack when I was near Mapleton. It got to be almost a family joke," she told me. Most of her attacks occurred where she lived and worked, but Mapleton, a quiet suburb about forty-five minutes from her home, seemed to have a mysterious triggering effect. Ellen had experienced many attacks there over the years. This was good evidence that her condition was due to stress illness because few, if any, other diseases would react so consistently to geography. Unfortunately, no other clues were readily available about what her body was trying to say about this precise location. There were no people, events, or other associations with Mapleton that were the least bit stressful for Ellen. With a shrug, she said, "I don't even know anyone who lives there."

Not ready to leave this clue behind, I introduced the possibility that stress played a role in causing her symptoms. Ellen accepted this premise and we began looking for sources of stress in her present life, or from depression, trauma, or anxiety, but she had no problems in these areas. Then we began talking about her childhood. Initially, she was reluctant to discuss her life before the onset of the illness, as if she wasn't sure why it was relevant. However, as she began answering my questions, a wealth of information poured forth. Ellen's parents had a bitter divorce when she was four years old. Compounding this difficulty was her mother's continued animosity toward her father. As a result, Ellen had almost no contact with him. To make matters worse, she resembled her father physically (father and daughter were both blonde, while her mother was dark-haired), and because of this her mother often displaced some of her anger onto Ellen. The situation became worse after her mother remarried and had children with Ellen's stepfather. These younger siblings received most of the parental attention, affection, gifts, and privileges while Ellen did the chores. As she put it: "I grew up like Cinderella, but without the Prince." Her self-esteem clearly suffered.

Admissions of hurt and anger colored Ellen's recollections as she told me that her mother's behavior hardly improved as Ellen became an adult. As she grew older, Ellen continued trying to ignore her feelings of resentment just as she had done as a child. "My attitude was I could not do anything to change my childhood," Ellen told me. She made an effort to let the past go and work toward a better relationship with her mother and stepfather.

In the meantime, other aspects of her life were going well. In addition to her fulfilling career, raising her children, and her marriage to an affectionate, hard-working man, Ellen made major strides in building self-esteem lost during childhood. At the same time, she badly wanted her mother's approval, and hoped that somehow, some way, her achievements would earn it. For years, she kept her resentment to herself, but it was evident to me that her conflicting feelings had become increasingly powerful. With this in mind, we returned to Mapleton. There had to be something there that increased the emotional pressure. If she did not know anybody in Mapleton, and she nearly always became ill in Mapleton, why did she go there?

"Well, it's on the way here," she explained. "We come to southern Washington about once a year, and Mapleton is on the way. That's the only reason."

My question: "Did you pass by Mapleton on your trip here this time?"
Ellen's answer: "Yes, last week, and I got sick then, too, but it only lasted for that day. I didn't need the hospital until I got sick again yesterday."

My question: "Is there any special reason why you drive here every year?"
Ellen's answer: "We come here to visit my mother and stepfather."

Suddenly, it became easy to imagine what might be happening during these journeys. Ellen would get in her car and begin thinking about the upcoming visit with her family. The prospect of enduring the same put-downs and insensitive treatment she had suffered throughout her life would cause increasing anguish as the car brought her closer to her parent's home. By the time she reached Mapleton, the tension level might be enough to make her physically ill. When presented with this idea, Ellen admitted it was possible, but was not completely convinced. I searched for a way to test the theory, pointing out that Mapleton was about forty-five minutes from her departure point. But, on her return trip, Ellen confirmed, she had never experienced an attack while driving forty-five minutes in the other direction. She also realized, when I asked her about it, that as long as she was not on her way to her parent's home, she could drive forty-five minutes in almost any direction without becoming ill.

This meant the only possible explanation for the many attacks in Mapleton was the emotional tension with her mother. For the first time, Ellen recognized the cause of her illness. She looked up at the ceiling and said, "Oh my God, I can't believe it!" Her husband, who had not said a word up to that point, was shaking his head in astonishment. He suddenly recalled that many of Ellen's attacks began soon after she spoke to her mother on the phone. Neither of them had recognized the significance of this coincidence.

From that moment, Ellen's illness was over. We spoke at length about how childhood stress can result in an adult disease. We addressed the power of emotional stress to produce physical illness, about how connections between the past and present can manifest, and how the mind can release suppressed anger into the body.

Ellen was now able to comprehend what her body had been trying to tell her. For the first time, the enormous emotional tension in the relationship with her mother reached the light of conscious awareness. After fifteen years, she finally had an alternative to expressing emotions through her body. In Ellen's case, being able to talk about her feelings relieved them enough that the physical illness ended on the spot. I followed up with some other treatment suggestions, including some I'll be discussing later on. The grand test came a year later when Ellen returned to southern Washington to visit her mother. She called me to report that her attacks had not returned, even when passing through Mapleton.

As you can see, the cause of Ellen's stress illness was easy to find. The answer should not have taken fifteen years to diagnose and probably not even fifteen days. After all, if an ulcer, a gallstone, or a brain tumor had caused her illness, then failure to diagnose it would be unforgivable. Failing to diagnose stress illness should be equally deplorable, but instead that failing is routine. How did Ellen end up in a blind spot in the health care system? First, doctors who evaluated her for visible physical disease did not know what to look for when her diagnostic tests were normal. Next, her psychiatrist did not know what to look for after determining she did not have a mental illness. Without the necessary training for health care professionals – already overburdened by large caseloads – there was no one who could ask the right questions and understand what to do with the answers. The result is that Ellen and millions like her fall into a large hole in the system.

Even after we have created institutional changes to solve this problem, it will still be up to individual doctors to listen more closely to what our patients' bodies are trying to tell us. That was a vital lesson I learned early in my career.

THE POWER OF LISTENING

As a kid growing up, I had a reputation for being a good listener and just seemed to be the kind of person other children confided in. Perhaps my curiosity about others began while living in Venezuela during pre-school and kindergarten. Traveling to a different land and experiencing a new culture was fascinating and seemed to carry over into wanting to learn who people were and what was happening in their lives. When I was nine, a girl I knew came to tell me about problems she was having at home. While my own family life was stable, supportive and relatively stress-free, it was apparent that other kids experienced significant problems. For them, I could do little more than listen and commiserate. In time, I came to see that in many situations the act of listening itself was enough to make a difference.

As I began my medical career, I learned that listening without judgment was essential in helping patients get well. My greatest satisfactions are in making a connection with others, understanding them, and promoting their self-understanding. As a physician, that's what I love most about what I do – those moments of mutual understanding between doctor and patient, when I can see the self-discovery in their eyes, when we nod simultaneously in agreement about a cause or consequence of a baffling illness, or when we find an effective treatment.

These doctor-to-patient exchanges played a key role in the growth of my knowledge of stress medicine. When I arrived in Portland, Oregon and started my work in internal medicine and gastroenterology at a large multi-specialty group, I brought with me the principles learned from an extraordinary mentor, Dr. Kaplan of UCLA. Because there were no mentors in Portland, and few scientific journal articles or textbooks available to continue formal study, I learned by listening to patients whom no one else could cure. Beginning in 1984, I interviewed up to four hundred stress illness patients annually for an hour each, which was usually enough time for them to trust me with their most difficult and painful experiences. I learned steadily, while also being aware of the risk of heading off into uncharted and potentially invalid medical practice. What kept me on track was the health of the patient. If she or he improved – and these patients had not made progress elsewhere in the health care system – then I knew I was on the right track. Early on, I often needed several visits with a patient to understand the source of their illness. After five or six years, I had diagnostic and therapeutic success with most patients during the initial encounter.

My fellow physicians acknowledged my progress with awards for the quality of my work, with referral of their most difficult cases and with requests for me to create teaching seminars on stress illness – for patients, health care professionals, and medical trainees. The increasing popularity of the seminars led to my publication of a brochure on stress illness that is available throughout my medical group's facilities in the Northwest. I share this success with every stress illness patient, for their true heroism in sharing personal stories with those of us working in this small but growing field. There is one patient, in particular, who deserves special recognition.

I met Catherine over twenty years ago while I was at UCLA. After four years of medical school, a year of internship, and two years of training in the diagnosis and treatment of diseases of adults, I was without any education pertaining to stress illness (just like nearly all other physicians). This meant I was wholly unprepared to help Catherine. We spent only an hour together, but the encounter completely changed my medical career.

At first, there seemed nothing unusual about Catherine. She was a forty-two-year-old mother of several children, slender with light brown hair, and happily married. She enjoyed her work as a part-time assistant in a law firm. Catherine told me she had been quite healthy until two years before when she developed severe abdominal pain and diarrhea alternating with constipation. Even with high doses of several medicines, the problems continued.

After eight doctors and numerous normal tests, she went to a university medical center. The evaluation there was completely normal. The specialized testing we offered at UCLA also showed nothing.

When I asked if she had been under a lot of stress recently, as other doctors had asked her, Catherine shrugged and replied, "Just the stress from being sick."

My next question was: "Were you under any stress earlier?" I was wondering if she had experienced a specific stress when her illness began two years before. She interpreted the question to mean the more remote past.

"Yes," she replied calmly and with little hesitation. "My father molested me."

This was the first time anyone had made this revelation to me and I had no idea how to respond. Without any childhood stress of my own to recall, or any medical training about how to relate this information to her illness, I was at a loss for words. Would it be better to ignore her statement? Would exploring this issue add emotional trauma to Catherine's medical condition? Why had she decided to reveal such a personal issue? My medical curiosity quickly became stronger than my fear of asking for more details. After all, we were at the absolute end with diagnostic tests, so there was not much to lose by delving further into her past. Besides, in the first month of medical school I had learned that you could take a patient's history even without knowing what to do with the information.

Catherine told me her earliest memory of her father molesting her was at age four. The molestation continued regularly for the next eight years. When she began menstruating, he stopped. There were no other incidents of abuse or personal trauma in her life. Was it possible for sexual abuse to cause illness in a healthy person thirty years later? The answer to that question is "yes, definitely," but on that day, I had no idea.

I then returned to my earlier question about whether a more recent event had triggered her symptoms. I asked whether anything difficult or negative had occurred just before her symptoms began. Catherine shook her head no. On the contrary, she replied, "The only thing I remember is that I quit working for this total jerk and got a new job where everyone is great." She had been with the difficult supervisor for ten years and felt liberated when she left.

Now I was even more confused. Could changing to a better job trigger a severe illness? (I learned later that the answer to that question is also "yes, definitely.") I could see no connection between any of these events and her illness. Moreover, she had received counseling about the sexual abuse long ago. Catherine had no symptoms of depression or other mental illness to suggest that a psychiatric evaluation would help but, fortunately, Dr. Kaplan, a member of our Psychiatry department who had extensive training in Internal Medicine as well, agreed to talk with her. Hoping Dr. Kaplan could find some answers, I explained to Catherine there was nothing more I could do. I watched her bravely leave the examination room, and that was the last I saw of her.

Four months later, I ran into Dr. Kaplan in an elevator and asked how Catherine was doing. "Well, I haven't seen her in over a month, Dave," she replied. "Her bowels are working just fine now." Catherine was no longer ill! She had even stopped taking the medicines I had recommended.

I exited the elevator in a mild state of shock and then turned to ask, "How did you do that?" as the elevator doors were closing between us. My medical training, typical for most students, never included the concept of alleviating a serious physical condition solely by counseling. Shortly thereafter, I had the wonderful opportunity to work with Dr. Kaplan again and begin my education about stress illness. Over the next few years, I learned everything I could from Dr. Kaplan and the many patients she helped with her remarkable insights into how human beings cope with stress. She taught me the differences between visible and invisible illnesses, what questions to ask patients and how to respond to the answers, and how to listen from both psychological and physiological perspectives. Soon I was able to help my patients in ways I had never imagined before.

The more I learned later on in my own practice, the better I understood the process that produced Catherine's symptoms. In a later chapter, I'll talk more about what I refer to as the "I Deserve Better" stage, which is a step on the way to getting past childhood stress but is a consequence of that stress as well. In Catherine's case, her illness began when she reached that stage. The sexual abuse from childhood had left her with poor self-esteem so, even as an adult, she put up with a verbally abusive supervisor for ten years. With the support of a loving husband, Catherine's personal growth led her to realize there was no reason to endure her toxic boss any longer. She decided she deserved a better job and had no difficulty finding work in a new, pleasant, and supportive environment.

With her new job, Catherine suddenly found herself appreciated at work as well as at home. Family, friends, and co-workers were unanimous in their affection for her. She recognized that her feelings of guilt, shame, and inadequacy were unjustified and began to see herself as positive and strong. She then recognized how wronged she had been as a little girl. There was anger, but she had learned while very young how to put such emotions into a box. From that box, the emotions traveled to her bowels and caused them to spasm uncontrollably.

Working with Dr. Kaplan, Catherine was able to find the emotions and put them into words. Together they pried open her box of rage and released the contents for feeling, thinking, writing, and speaking. In just a few months, Catherine's stress illness symptoms completely disappeared.

In addition to lessons about the power of listening learned from every one of the seven thousand heroic patients who have trusted me with their most difficult personal challenges, I learned another vital lesson that might run counter to other approaches to stress you might have read or heard about. Contrary to some popular self-help approaches, and clearly shown by the stories of Ellen and Catherine, healing stress illness cannot be done simply by making lifestyle changes in the absence of understanding the causes of the illness. *Identification and understanding of the hidden forces that conspire to undermine progress is fundamental to reaching a person's full potential for healing.* However, before we start looking at those forces in detail and the treatment options that can help, let us look at a question that might well be on your mind now.

COULD YOU HAVE STRESS ILLNESS?

Symptoms of stress illness can strike anywhere in your body. Why they occur in one location and not another is usually unclear. Some patients have just one of the symptoms we will be talking about and some have more. One recent patient of mine had fifteen distinct symptoms and another handed me a printed list of twenty-seven symptoms he was experiencing. (The more symptoms a person has, the more likely it is that stress illness is the underlying cause.) When medical tests are negative or inconclusive, you have good reason to explore the possibility of stress illness with your doctor, using this book as a guide.

> As we discuss the common symptoms of stress illness throughout this book, please remember that many other diseases can cause these symptoms. Until your illness is gone, it is essential that you work with a qualified doctor to determine if a condition other than stress illness is responsible.

The most common symptom of stress illness is pain. This can occur almost anywhere in the body and often in more than one location at a time. Some common stress-related pains are headache, pain or stiffness in the joint of the upper jaw, back pain, or chest pain. Chest pain can resemble the pressure of a heart attack or feel like an ache or burning sensation. Pain and stiffness of the neck and shoulders or anywhere in the spine is also common.

Pain in the abdomen or reproductive organs can be highly variable in location and timing from day to day. The pain can also be constant. It can be in one small area or throughout the abdomen and pelvis or anywhere in between. With the pain, there can be constipation or diarrhea or these two symptoms can alternate with each other. Constipation or diarrhea can also occur without any pain. (However, stress illness does not cause bleeding in the gastrointestinal tract.) Other digestion-related symptoms that can occur in stress illness include gagging, swallowing problems, a sensation of a lump in the throat, indigestion, lack of appetite, cramping, bloating, "gas" sensation, nausea, vomiting, and rectal pain.

Respiratory tract problems that can be due to stress illness include difficulty breathing (either all the time or just occasionally), a recurring cough, or changes in the voice. Stress can also cause nerve symptoms such as feeling faint, dizziness, ringing in the ears, itching of the skin, and numbness or tingling in the hands or feet.

Any of these symptoms can be present for a few seconds at a time or persist almost constantly for decades. They can occur in almost any combination. Sometimes a pain will stop after a surgical procedure only to return after weeks, months, or years. Occasionally the pain will stop in the part of the body that had surgery, but re-emerge somewhere else.

Before referral to me, one patient had pain in the right side of her pelvis until she had surgery to remove her right ovary. Some time later pain re-occurred in the mid-pelvis. Removal of her uterus gave relief. After she felt well for a time, pain returned in the left side of her pelvis and she had her left ovary surgically removed. She was again temporarily well until pain returned in the lower left abdomen. This last pain was relieved after discovery and treatment of significant lifelong stress issues. Since her female organs were normal when a pathologist examined them after each surgery, I suspected that her previous pains were due to the same stress.

If you have one or more of the symptoms described in this chapter, how can you tell if stress is the cause? Try using the following three steps.

1. Get an evaluation by your doctor. If this is normal then it is much more likely (but not proven) that stress is responsible for the symptom.

2. Make a list of sources of stress in your life that might be capable of causing illness. This is a key step in understanding everything you might be coping with. Many people are aware of the existence of stressful issues, but do not fully appreciate the degree of difficulty they are causing. In many interviews, my patients initially denied experiencing excessive stress only to recognize later that they were coping with much more than they thought. Making the list will help you comprehend your burdens more accurately. Further understanding will come from reading detailed descriptions of the five different types of stress in the pages just ahead. Finally, you will gain even more insights from the stories in Part II.

3. Apply the seven key principles we will discuss for reducing or eliminating the causes and consequences of the stress. If these techniques lead to relief of your symptoms then you can have a lot of confidence that the stress caused the illness.

By now, you might be curious about how stress can literally make you sick. For the answer, a brief explanation of the stress response system is in order.

IN THE ABSENCE OF PREDATORS

Begin by imagining that millions of years ago, one of your ancestors was picking berries when she observed a hungry saber-tooth cat emerging from the bushes. In her brain, a series of interconnected areas called the stress response system kicked into high gear to help her cope. Another name for this is the "fight or flight" system because it mobilizes the body to face danger head on or to run away. This system operates in many species to coordinate the response to predators and other threats. The human stress response apparatus sent nerve signals into your ancestor's body and caused her heart to beat faster, muscles to tense, breathing to become more rapid, sweat to appear, and digestive and bowel function to slow. These changes helped her survive the confrontation, which is why we need a stress response system in our bodies.

Human beings are no longer confronting saber-tooth cats, but the stresses we face today can still trigger the stress response system. Running a race, speaking in public, taking a chemistry exam (my personal saber-tooth cat), walking into an important job interview, fighting with your mother, going on a first date, or having a dispute with a neighbor can all cause stress. Happy occasions such as the birth of a child, the purchase of a new home, getting married, or winning an award can cause stress too. The resulting "butterflies in the stomach," fast and shallow breathing, muscle tension, rapid heartbeat, or sweating palms are experiences common to us all. These physical responses are part of our preparation for maximum effort.

It is important to recognize that some stresses last for just a short time, others for much longer. For example, imagine you are driving down a residential street. A small child darts in front of your vehicle. You see the child and your brain calculates the danger. Your stress response system surges into action. Nerve signals race into your body, enabling you to apply the brakes quickly and forcefully. The child is unharmed. In this case, the stress is over in a short time. The nerve signals from the stress response system stop and the body returns to its usual state, so there are no long-lasting consequences.

Prolonged stress, on the other hand, can cause problems for the body. When the nerve signals from the stress response center persist, the body is unable to return to an unstressed state. For example, imagine you are living with someone who loses his or her temper often or hits you. You are never sure when you might be threatened, so there is stress whenever that person is present. Most of the time the level of stress is not as high as in the previous example, but it is present for a much longer period. For our purposes, it is convenient to assume that *the physical symptoms of stress illness occur when nerve signals from the stress response system persist for too long at too high a level.*

Symptoms that result from this process can be indistinguishable from those caused by other diseases. They can be mild or severe and can occur almost anywhere in the body. In one of my patients, the strongest nerve signals from the stress response system went to the stomach. Her illness began with abdominal "butterflies." Over time, her stress became worse and the nerve signals strengthened. Her condition progressed to nausea, then vomiting and finally complete paralysis of the stomach. Finding a solution to her stress stopped the nerve signals and her stomach returned to normal.

The nerve signals rarely cause damage to the body's organs. This is why diagnostic tests are nearly always normal. One of my patients was ill for over *eighty years* and her diagnostic tests still showed no physical abnormalities. Of course, this causes a major dilemma for doctors who usually are unable to "find anything wrong" and the patient becomes a medical mystery.

Fortunately, as we have seen with Ellen and Catherine, the diagnosis of stress illness does not depend on tests, but rather on understanding the patient as a person. The diagnostic process can then begin with a search for stresses capable of causing illness.

It is worth repeating that many doctors are reluctant to mention the possibility that a patient's symptoms could be due to stress. This is because patients often resent any implication that symptoms are "in their head" or in any way imaginary. This is why I emphasize that stress causes symptoms just as real as those of any other disease. As physicians, we can remind our patients that the symptoms of stress illness are due to nerve signals from the brain similar to those that help us react to sudden threats — a real process that has operated in all human beings since we became a species.

Another tool for understanding how this might apply to you, is the diagram below. The arrows from "Stress" to the brain illustrate difficult life events arriving at the stress response system for processing. For our purposes, it is reasonable to assume that if the level of incoming stress is excessive, this system can unload stress into the body in the form of nerve impulses. When these signals are strong enough, they can cause symptoms. The location of the symptoms depends on where the signals go in the body. In this diagram, you can see the impulses emerging from the nervous system and traveling into many areas of the body.

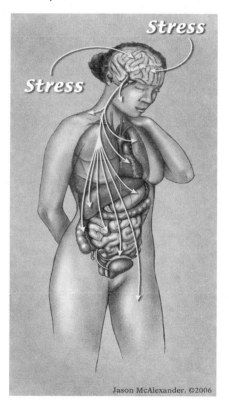

Jason McAlexander, ©2006

Now that you understand the stress response process, your next step is to determine what stresses in your life might be strong enough to trigger this reaction in your body.

THE FIVE TYPES OF STRESS

Difficult, frightening, or emotionally painful experiences occur in almost everyone's life and many of them are capable of causing stress illness. There is great diversity in these illness-causing conditions, but they tend to fall into five categories. The categories are:

- Childhood stress
- Stress occurring now
- Stress from a traumatic event
- Stress from depression, a mental health condition
- Stress from an anxiety disorder, a mental health condition

As you look at the descriptions that follow, bear in mind that the categories tend to overlap and events in one category can influence the response to events in another.

Childhood Stress. One of the biggest surprises of my medical career was learning that stress in childhood is often a cause of illness in adults. Childhood stress comes from experiences that lower self-esteem in a child for a prolonged period. Often the low self-esteem persists well into the adult years. These problems can result when a child experiences one or more of the following:

- Being frequently hit, slapped, kicked, or beaten
- Recurring shame, ridicule, mocking, or being made fun of by family or peers
- Repeatedly being made to feel that nothing they do is ever good enough
- Genital fondling, sexual intercourse, or other forms of sexual abuse

- Neglect with respect to affection, emotional support, safety, shelter, clothing, or food
- Witnessing violence
- Parental abuse of drugs or alcohol
- Being given responsibilities not appropriate for a child
- Fear of real or potential danger in their home or neighborhood

An important study from the University of Washington focusing on pain in the female pelvis illustrates the connection between stress in childhood and physical symptoms in adults. The subjects of this study were two groups of women undergoing laparoscopy (pronounced "lap ah ross kah pee"), a surgical procedure in which a metal tube with a camera examines the interior of the abdomen or pelvis. All the women in the first group had severe pelvic pain. In the second group, none of the women had pain but they needed the laparoscopy because they had been unable to become pregnant.

Most of the women in both groups had normal laparoscopy examinations. Some women with pain had abnormalities such as scar tissue, cysts on their ovaries, or endometriosis (tissue from the lining of the uterus that had leaked out and grown in the pelvis). It would be natural to assume, as many doctors do, that these problems were the cause of the pain. However, the research discovered that the women who had no pain had these abnormalities just as often. Why should scar tissue, for example, that looked the same in two women, cause severe pain in one and no pain at all in another? Perhaps the scar tissue and the other abnormalities were not the cause of the pain after all.

These results raised two questions. First, what was causing the pain if the cysts, scar tissue, or endometriosis was not causing it? Second, what was causing the pain in the women who had normal laparoscopies? The answer to both questions might be stress illness. The researchers uncovered an intriguing clue that suggests a link between the pain and childhood stress. They asked all the women in both groups about sexual abuse prior to the age of fifteen. Of the women experiencing chronic pelvic pain, sixty-four percent had experienced some degree of sexual abuse. Of the women with no pain, twenty-one percent had experienced sexual abuse, which is average (unfortunately) for adult American women. In other words, *sexual abuse in childhood occurred three times as often among adult women with unexplained pelvic pain as it did among women without pain.*

This evidence is not conclusive proof that sexual abuse in childhood was the cause of the pain that occurred many years later in these women. There could be another cause not yet discovered. However, it does illustrate a strong association between a particular childhood stress and unexplained pain in adults. This association is common in my practice where over half of my stress illness patients have experienced significant childhood stress of one sort or another, not necessarily related to sexual abuse.

This study illustrates another common issue in stress illness patients, the problem of diagnostic tests finding abnormalities that have nothing to do with a patient's symptoms. In this study, few if any women had pain caused by endometriosis, cysts, or adhesions. Yet when doctors detect an abnormality in the body near the location of the symptoms, it is very easy to conclude that the abnormality is the cause. I have cared for hundreds of patients after removal of an appendix, ovary, uterus, or gallbladder who found that their pain persisted until someone investigated their stresses.

Stress Occurring Now. As the second type of stress frequently capable of causing illness, stress occurring in a person's life right now can be purely personal (such as a mid-life crisis) or involve other people in the family or workplace. Substance abuse, family disputes, marital discord, violence from an intimate partner, financial problems, workplace harassment, persistent lack of personal time, and death of a loved one are all capable of producing stress illness.

Having a medical illness can also be a stress that contributes to symptoms of stress illness. Sometimes the medical disease and stress illness cause completely different symptoms. In other cases, the medical condition and the stress condition cause the same symptom. This is a particularly difficult diagnostic challenge. One example is a patient who had an inflammatory condition of her bowel that caused diarrhea. She also had a severe stress that caused diarrhea. It was only when both problems were treated that her diarrhea stopped. Later, in Part Two, the chapter on multi-factorial stresses will address diagnosis and treatment when visible disease and stress illness occur together.

Stress from a Traumatic Event. The third type of stress, experienced at some time in the lives of ten percent of the population, is a traumatic event. Surviving an assault or serious accident, being in military combat, witnessing violence, or enduring the unanticipated or violent death of a loved one can cause stress that can be short term or of much longer duration.

In some cases, these events cause a condition known as post-traumatic stress disorder (PTSD). Symptoms of PTSD include:

- Distressing memories of the trauma that intrude into your thoughts
- Nightmares related to the trauma
- Flashbacks where you might feel you are reliving the trauma
- Strong emotional reactions to any reminders of the trauma
- Disturbed sleep patterns
- Emotional numbness and loss of pleasure in life
- Easy startling
- Frequent irritability or anger

The physical symptoms of stress illness, such as pain or altered bowel function, are common in those recovering from a traumatic event. These physical symptoms can occur even when the symptoms of post-traumatic stress disorder are not prominent.

Depression. The fourth type of stress comes from the mental health condition doctors call depression. This disorder usually responds well to treatment and is not difficult to diagnose in patients who:

- Feel depressed, down or hopeless
- Cry frequently for no obvious reason
- Feel profound fatigue

- Believe that life is no longer worth living and that death might be preferable to their emotional pain (if you feel this way, contact a doctor immediately)

However, most patients with depression do not have such straightforward symptoms. They might not feel depressed or suicidal. Instead, they might notice:

- Difficulty falling asleep or difficulty remaining asleep through the night
- Loss of interest or pleasure in activities they formerly enjoyed
- Reduced interest in food, sometimes causing loss of weight (A smaller number of patients with depression eat more and therefore might gain weight.)
- Less ability to cope with normal day-to-day stresses
- Lower general energy
- Feelings of worthlessness or guilt
- Difficulty concentrating

Depression can reveal itself with some or all of the above symptoms. This disorder can become severe enough to produce stress illness even when there are no other obvious stresses present. This surprises many of my patients. "How can I be depressed?" they wonder. "I have no reason to be depressed, my life is fine!" In these cases, depression results from a chemical imbalance in the nervous system that might have little to do with life experiences.

In other patients, depression co-exists with and magnifies stress from one or more of the other four categories (childhood, past trauma, problems in current life, anxiety). At the same time, these other stresses can make the depression worse. A vicious cycle can result as depression reduces the ability to cope, making other life stresses more difficult to manage which then worsens the depression.

Anxiety Disorders. This fifth type of stress is also a mental health condition that usually responds well to treatment. There are several types, but in all of them patients have excessive fears or dread out of proportion to any cause. For example, it is appropriate to feel anxious if a stranger approaches while you are alone in a dark parking lot. Feeling that same degree of anxiety while with friends at a restaurant could be due to an anxiety disorder.

The extreme of anxiety disorders is a panic attack. This episode of overwhelming anxiety, fear, or terror has no clear (i.e. conscious) reason for it to occur. Panic attacks generally occur with no warning, can happen at any time of day or night, reach their peak within minutes, and are often associated with one or more of the following physical symptoms:

- Rapid heartbeat
- Sweating
- Difficulty breathing
- Lightheadedness
- Numbness or tingling of the hands, feet or lips
- Abdominal or chest pain
- Feeling like you are dying

When these physical symptoms are more prominent than the fear or dread, doctors might not consider panic as a possible cause while they look for an abnormality in the body. Medical conditions that can sometimes cause similar symptoms include an overactive thyroid, abnormal electrical rhythms in the heart, excessive use of stimulants (caffeine and decongestants are two common examples), and, rarely, tumors that secrete large amounts of the hormone adrenaline. Correct diagnosis of panic attacks might not occur for several years if doctors fail to consider it as a possibility.

When panic attacks occur repeatedly, doctors then call the condition panic disorder. Anxiety about when and where the next episode will occur can develop. Patients then avoid certain locations and situations in which previous attacks took place. Since panic can occur anywhere and at any time, some individuals will end up avoiding so much that they lead very restricted lives. Some people have so much difficulty coping with this disorder that they become depressed or turn to street drugs or alcohol for relief.

Another form of anxiety disorder is generalized anxiety. In this condition, the patient does not have panic attacks, but is anxious or worried most of the time. The anxiety lasts for many months or years and disrupts lives by interfering with the ability to relax, to concentrate, to sleep, or to enjoy life.

In social anxiety disorder, the patient experiences fear of embarrassment or judgment by others. The trigger for this is one or more types of social situations such as public speaking, eating with other people, or simply being with large numbers of people. As with the other anxiety disorders, the degree of fear or anxiety is out of proportion to the situation, is not easily controlled and interferes with the patient's life.

For every stress illness patient, finding and treating the underlying cause – childhood stress, current stress, traumatic stress, depression, anxiety, or a combination of these – is essential to helping them become well. It is important to acknowledge that for some patients this process requires years of work, often with a mental health counselor in addition to a primary care clinician. It is common to be unable to cope with some or all stress issues right away. Nevertheless, with perseverance, even the most difficult situations can improve.

AN OVERVIEW OF THE SEVEN KEYS TO HEALING STRESS ILLNESS

As mentioned earlier, it is vital to employ these principles in collaboration with a health care professional who has ruled out visible illnesses with diagnostic tests. As you work with your doctor, and particularly if you approach the point where "they can't find anything wrong," these seven keys to uncovering and managing "what's eating you" will start you on the road to recovery in the same way they have served thousands of my patients who overcame stress illness. They are explained briefly here, and there is an expanded discussion of these principles in a later chapter.

Key 1 – Understand that your symptoms can be diagnosed and treated. Just because physicians cannot find the source of your illness does not mean you are a hypochondriac or your symptoms are imaginary. It is not in your head! Stress illness symptoms are just as real as symptoms caused by any other disease and just as amenable to diagnosis and treatment. The only difference is that diagnosis does not depend on blood tests and scans.

Key 2 – Search for the sources of stress. Imagine you are a detective preparing to sift through evidence that includes the frequency and location of your symptoms and any connections you can find to the events of your life. Continue your detective work by creating an inventory of stresses past and present. Read about the characteristic symptoms of depression, post-traumatic stress, and anxiety to see if any apply to you. Look for connections in the evidence as you listen closely to what your body is telling you. In the pages ahead, the stories of how others have discovered clues and cures will give you insights.

Key 3 – Care for yourself. Symptoms can be the body's way of telling you to care for yourself. Self-care appears to be a simple recommendation but my patients often struggle with hidden forces that undermine their best intentions. In the chapters ahead, you will study these challenges and learn techniques for overcoming them.

Key 4 – Get right by writing. Many of the stories coming up illustrate the amazing therapeutic value of verbalizing trapped feelings – either through spoken words or by putting words on paper. Physical symptoms often result from the brain sending trapped emotions into the body. Converting the suppressed feelings into words provides the brain with a different outlet. For many patients, the more emotions they can express verbally, the less the brain will need to unload into the body. Writing, even more than speaking, has a way of revealing thoughts and emotions people did not suspect they had.

Key 5 – Employ appropriate therapies. Several effective therapies for stress illness involve collaboration between patients and health care professionals. Physicians can prescribe medications, refer to a mental health counselor, or both, or recommend forms of group counseling specific to the type of stress involved. You will read about these in the pages ahead and we will also discuss the help some patients find from religious counseling, prayer, and spiritual support.

Key 6 – Overcome hidden resistance. This principle will help you understand why and how stress illness might be resistant to treatment or subject to recurrence. You will learn about veiled forces that can undermine your strongest efforts and best intentions to manage stress. These factors can significantly diminish the benefits of well-intended advice about lifestyle changes for stress reduction. Identifying and coping with these issues will help you overcome barriers to wellness.

Key 7 – Become the person you were always meant to be. Using the first six keys will reveal the stresses you are dealing with and the factors that limit your ability to respond to these challenges. As you overcome these problems, you will develop a deeper and more accurate understanding of yourself. Pride in having survived those challenges will replace frustration. This personal growth will enhance your self-esteem, improve your ability to care for yourself, and facilitate managing anything life confronts you with in the future.

Of thousands of patients I have treated in my practice, most appear to return to healthy, fulfilling lives. Many reclaim not only their health, but their zest for life and their ability to become the person they were always meant to be. You will see this in the many case histories that follow and as you explore embracing life beyond the limitations of stress illness.

USING THIS BOOK

As I listen to a patient in my office, their story connects to others I have heard over the years. This helps me to answer the question "Hello, who are you?" and to find the stress or stresses that are most likely responsible for their symptoms. A principal challenge for this book is to help the reader who has not heard thousands of stress illness stories. How do I help someone to help herself or himself if they know only their own story? Another challenge is that most people with stress illness are not fully aware of the underlying stress. How do I help that person find and understand the key stress or stresses?

My answer to these questions is to provide a collection of stories large enough to illustrate a broad spectrum of stress illness. These case histories form the heart of the next six chapters. They will point out hidden stresses that caused physical symptoms in other patients. Then, if you suffer from stress illness, you can provide your health care professional with my recommended exercises and treatment recommendations. This will add to your understanding and provide new options on your path toward healing.

Professionals in diagnostic medicine, surgery, and mental health also can use the book to help close the gaps in our health care system that have failed millions of patients with stress illness. Ideally, the information here will be a foundation for more collaboration between patients, caregivers, doctors, mental health therapists and policymakers in the health care system. Above all, I hope the stories of my heroic patients will inspire you, as they do me.

CHAPTER 2

HELLO. WHO ARE YOU?

Definition of a normal person: "Someone you don't know very well."

– Anonymous

THE DIAGNOSIS OF STRESS ILLNESS DEPENDS ON UNDERSTANDING THE WHOLE person, often including the patient's childhood experience. As we saw earlier with Ellen, much of this can be accomplished during the initial meeting between patient and physician. The key question for the patient at this early stage is – "Hello. Who are you?" The five stories in this chapter and those later on will help you identify key experiences in your life that have shaped who you are and might have laid the foundation for stress illness.

Then the next question, which you might ask yourself or a doctor might ask you is – "What is happening in your life now that could be connected to your symptoms?" The stories will give you insights into this question also.

A STARTING PLACE: WORKING WITH DOCTORS

Yolanda was a sixteen-year-old native of Guatemala with a beautiful but expressionless face. Her story demonstrates how doctors differ in their approach to patients with stress illness. Understanding this will help you work more effectively with a doctor as your partner.

When I teach groups of young doctors about Yolanda, I describe how she came to the medical walk-in clinic complaining of three weeks of episodes of blurred vision lasting for up to an hour. I then ask the doctors to pretend Yolanda is before them, ready for evaluation. The doctors ask questions about symptoms, about Yolanda's physical examination and about the results of laboratory tests and x-rays as they search for a diagnosis. Only a few doctors are able to track down the cause of her problem. To illustrate how some doctors help Yolanda and others do not, I will show you how Dr. Smith fails to find the correct diagnosis and how Dr. Jones succeeds. As a young doctor, I practiced a lot more like Dr. Smith than I usually care to admit.

Dr. Smith hears Yolanda describe her symptoms and immediately begins thinking about possible causes. He wonders whether her visual problems are part of a more widespread disease. Before Yolanda has had thirty seconds to tell her story, he interrupts with a number of questions to determine if she has had any other eye problems or nerve symptoms.

He learns Yolanda has had no symptoms of any kind except the blurred vision. Unfortunately, by interrupting with so many questions, Dr. Smith has given Yolanda the impression he has heard all he needs to about her symptoms. She keeps other issues that were on her mind to herself.

Yolanda's eye chart test is normal because she is not having blurred vision at the time of the visit. Dr. Smith then conducts the physical examination, which is normal except for a large bruise on the left side of her neck. Yolanda explains that one week before coming to the clinic, she said something to her mother that her father interpreted as disrespectful. He grabbed Yolanda by the throat so hard he caused the bruise and then threw her against the wall.

Dr. Smith focuses on the potential significance of this injury for Yolanda's vision. He knows that if she struck the back of her head when thrown against the wall this could affect the visual part of her brain. He is able to dismiss this possibility because there was no bruise on the back of the head, she did not lose consciousness, the incident took place two weeks after the blurred vision started and her vision was no worse afterward. He does not concern himself with the bruise any further.

Dr. Smith is uncertain about the cause of Yolanda's visual symptoms. He is concerned about nerve, brain or eye disease not detected by his examination. He orders blood tests, an MRI scan of her brain and a consultation with an eye specialist. These tests detect no abnormalities. Her blurred vision continues to come and go several times each week. Dr. Smith now cannot imagine that a nerve, brain or eye problem is causing the symptoms. Like many doctors, he is not experienced in evaluating for stress illness and is not sure what to do next. He tells Yolanda he "can't find anything wrong."

Dr. Jones takes a different approach. After hearing Yolanda's symptoms, Dr. Jones also forms hypotheses about possible causes, but she waits for Yolanda to finish talking before asking any questions. Yolanda seems to go off on a tangent, reviewing a number of problems in her home that are distressing to her. Among other issues, she mentions that her father has been "bothering her."

When Yolanda is finished, Dr. Jones asks the same questions that Dr. Smith asked and conducts the same eye chart test and physical examination. When she sees the injury to Yolanda's neck and hears how it happened, she remembers Yolanda's feelings of distress about her home. Dr. Jones now considers the possibility that stress illness is responsible for the blurred vision. She thinks about how to assess Yolanda's stresses in more detail.

Dr. Jones suspects that if Yolanda's father grasped her by the throat (causing a bruise that lasted for a week) and then threw her against a wall, other incidents of abuse could have occurred. She asks if the father has injured her at other times. Yolanda replies that similar abuse has occurred repeatedly during the last ten years.

This leads Dr. Jones to consider that Yolanda might be depressed. She learns that Yolanda suffers from interrupted sleep, severe fatigue, poor appetite and loss of pleasure in life. She has no plans to kill herself, but has thought about it.

Suddenly, a question occurs to Dr. Jones: when Yolanda's vision was blurred, did she notice if tears were running down her cheeks at those times? Yolanda remembered that she always had tears when her vision was blurred.

The cause of Yolanda's visual symptoms was crying. This was a result of her depression, which came from years of physical abuse. Child abuse survivors learn to stuff their anguish into a mental box, which shields them from much of the emotional pain. One consequence of this for Yolanda was that, with her misery stuffed away, she could not connect the physical response of crying with the emotion of sadness. Therefore, she could not perceive the crying for what it was, reacting to it instead only as blurred vision.

Dr. Jones arranged for an immediate visit with a social worker experienced in managing child abuse issues. The social worker explained to Yolanda that the abuse was going to stop. The subsequent intervention in her family was successful and Yolanda's depression and crying improved tremendously. Her visual problems stopped.

Evaluating a new patient can be like sorting through a pile of jigsaw pieces without having the completed picture as a guide. The path to the final image often includes many false starts and incorrect assumptions. Dr. Jones was successful because she gave Yolanda time to tell her story and did not focus solely on finding a visible disease to explain the symptom. Dr. Jones listened patiently to information that seemed irrelevant initially, but later turned out to be essential and enabled Dr. Jones to answer the question: "Hello, who are you?" Drs. Smith and Jones represent opposite ends of a spectrum of medical practice. Most doctors will fall somewhere in the middle in their management of stress illness. With this in mind, there are a number of ways in which you can help any doctor to help you.

To begin with, insist on presenting your most important concerns before the doctor begins their evaluation. Examples of these include new physical symptoms, serious stresses in your life or worries that you might have cancer or heart disease. You might want to write down all your concerns before the appointment. Then, if you have, say, three items on your list, a good way to start the conversation with your doctor would be "I have three concerns that I want to talk to you about today." Being clear about the number of issues you have will help you express your full agenda before the doctor begins her assessment. Try to be reasonable about the number of issues you present at any one visit. Doctors are busy, but most are comfortable managing two or three problems in one visit and saving others for a follow-up appointment.

Be prepared for the doctor who rapidly interrupts you to ask specific questions about your symptoms. These questions are essential, but it is perfectly acceptable to ask the doctor to wait until after you have shared all your concerns. Yolanda's interview with Dr. Smith did not include any of the crucial information about her home life or depression. Had she insisted on sharing the distress she felt about her home and communicated about her sleep disruption, fatigue and suicidal thoughts, Dr. Smith might have been in a much better position to help her.

For each of your symptoms, inform your doctor about when they began, how often they occur, how long they last, their exact location in your body, anything that seems to improve or worsen them and any ideas you have about what might be causing them. If you have had the same or similar symptom in the past then mention that too. If you have noticed a connection between your symptoms and one or more sources of stress, tell that to the doctor. As you read further in this book about the symptoms of childhood stress, current stress, depression, anxiety and post-traumatic stress, you can communicate these to your doctor if you have them.

Bring a list of all the medicines you take regularly. Include supplements, herbal treatments and non-prescription medicines such as pain relievers and cold remedies. Be sure to inform your doctor if you are using tobacco, alcohol or illegal drugs. If you have had a medical evaluation for your symptom(s) in the past, try to obtain a copy to bring to your doctor.

If you believe stress might be a factor in your symptoms, ask about resources available to help with the specific stresses you are coping with. If these prove to be useful, your symptoms could improve which will make you and your doctor more confident that stress is the cause. For example, suppose your illness began soon after the death of a loved one. Your doctor might be able to put you in touch with an expert in counseling about bereavement. If you find that your illness improves with this counseling then your doctor can use that information, combined with the results of diagnostic tests, to make better decisions about the need for any additional tests or treatments.

These techniques are intended to help you get the most out of your partnership with your physician. Stress illness is rarely easy to diagnose or treat, but persistence, patience and the ideas discussed in this book will help you find relief. See the box below for a summary checklist for working with doctors.

Checklist for Working with Doctors

- Try to bring records of previous medical evaluations of your condition.

- Write a list of your major concerns, trying for no more than four items.

- Insist on presenting all your major concerns, preferably before your doctor begins questioning you. Start by saying: "Doctor, I have _____ concerns to talk to you about today" (and fill in the blank with a number).

- Be sure to mention any symptoms of depression, anxiety or post-traumatic stress.

- For physical symptoms, describe their location, timing (when they began, how often they occur, any connection to stress) and factors that relieve or worsen the symptom.

- Bring a list of all your medicines (including non-prescription medicines, herbs and supplements) and tell your doctor if you are using tobacco, alcohol or illegal drugs.

- If you are struggling with one or more stresses, ask the doctor about resources that could help you.

Make sure to follow your doctor's recommendations. If you find you cannot do this for any reason, let the doctor know. Often doctors can find useful alternatives to their initial plan when something is not working for you.

As we saw earlier with Ellen and Catherine, dialogue with a physician can uncover powerful clues to diagnosing and treating stress illness by revealing who you are and what your life experiences have been. Other areas of potential interest will be the links between past and present stresses, connections between your self-esteem and personal stress and how belief systems from outside and within could be producing negative or positive consequences. The stories ahead in this chapter will help you understand these concepts. You will see how your identity – who you are, what you believe, what has happened in your life – plays a central role in your reaction to stress. Then, in Part II, we will explore each of the five types of stress in more depth followed by a more detailed look at the seven keys to healing. John's story below will introduce some of these ideas and show how they can help overcome even the most challenging of stress illnesses.

JOHN: SYMPTOMS SCRATCH THE SURFACE BUT CAUSES LIE DEEPER

John was a sixty-year-old retailer who sat in the exam room chair like a coiled spring, his fists resting motionless on his knees. Having attended one of my monthly classes on stress-related illness, he came to an individual appointment hoping for help with his peculiar itching. His concerned wife, Helen, came with him.

The problem began three years earlier and defied all attempts at diagnosis and treatment. John's itching occurred nearly every day, but might turn up in a different area of his body each time. One day the itching bothered him across his chest, the next day his hands, the next between his shoulder blades. Often it began in the evening, but occasionally after breakfast, too. The itching might last for minutes or hours.

I have never encountered a symptom remotely like this in another patient. His illness was so unusual that I was convinced stress was the cause. However, he had no stress in his life at the moment, no depression or anxiety, no history of trauma and no abuse as a child. I was at a loss to find questions that might help me understand his illness. I wanted to say, "John, your symptoms are very uncommon and a dermatologist and a neurologist have not been able to help you, so it isn't likely that I can help you either." While I was thinking this, he glared at the wall beside me. As my silence went on, he leaned forward in his chair like a football player waiting for the snap of the ball.

Something was about to be revealed, I was certain. So instead of giving up, I tried to learn who he was by encouraging him to talk about his life, allowing me to watch for clues as if they were jigsaw puzzle pieces appearing on a table. If I found enough pieces, the picture of his illness might become clearer. From patients like John, I have learned that when emotions are powerful enough to cause physical symptoms, the mind can usually find a way to express them to a listener who is open-minded and supportive. This can happen even when the speaker is not consciously aware of the source of the symptoms.

After I asked John to talk more about his life, starting with his childhood, he had no trouble opening up. His young life had not been easy. As a child, John received little in the way of emotional support. No one seemed to care about him much. He tried to earn affection by working hard for his family. He recalled chopping a cord of logs for the wood stove despite an injured back.

His long search for someone who would care for him came to a successful conclusion when he met Helen. He turned to smile at her with obvious affection, noting they had been together for four decades (and counting). Fifteen years earlier, John had almost lost her when a motor vehicle accident put her into intensive care for several days. She made a full recovery, but it was the most frightening time of their marriage.

Three years before coming to my office, John had another scare when he thought he might lose Helen again. She developed a liver disorder that caused steadily worsening jaundice accompanied by severe itching. Medical treatment did not seem to help. As the liver problem became more serious, a sense of dread came over John. He had a deep religious faith and, when there seemed almost no hope, prayed fervently for her to recover.

Just as I nodded to acknowledge the value of prayer, his next sentence provided the diagnosis for his illness. "I asked The Lord to let Helen live," he confided, "and that if she did He could give me her itching."

Soon after, one of my colleagues gave Helen a new treatment and the liver disease began to improve. After several months, the jaundice and itching healed completely. But both parts of John's prayer were answered: Helen recovered and he developed the itching.

We talked for a while. Then our conversation stopped as I tried to find words that might help John recover. I tried to imagine how John perceived his life and loved ones. John's family neglected him emotionally as a child. Helen came into his life like a rescue ship to a man lost at sea. He felt far closer to Helen than most husbands feel toward their wives. The possibility of her death bordered on terrifying. His prayer for a cure was the most heartfelt of his life. After her recovery, John remained fearful her disease might return. It would not be surprising if he were searching for reassurance this would not happen.

Perhaps, I suggested, a part of him believed the itching meant God was still answering his prayer and still protecting Helen. "And," I wondered aloud, "if the itching ever stopped, you might be afraid that her liver disease would return." Helen's mouth opened in surprise as she turned to John to see how he would respond.

John considered my idea and replied, "Dr. Clarke, I think you may have hit the nail on the head."

Until that moment, he had not been consciously aware of this possibility or even the connection between the itching and his prayer. I suggested that after three years he might have suffered enough in return for his wife's recovery. Nodding tentatively, John agreed that this seemed reasonable and he would think about it. Over the next several weeks, he accepted what Helen's doctors told him years before: her illness probably would never return, but if it did the same treatment would again be successful. John was then able to let go of most of his fear for Helen's health. When I called a month later, his itching was nearly gone.

Giving John a chance to tell his story revealed the hidden cause of the itching. This allowed John to use his faith to overcome fear of loss and fear of the unknown. After three long years, he found relief. My patient Rachel, as you will read next, suffered from stress illness for decades. The power of telling her story had a similarly transformational effect.

IT'S NEVER TOO LATE TO HEAL: RACHEL

Rachel did not have a fond image of the Kansas farmhouse where she was born in 1905. In those small wooden rooms, she suffered repeated beatings from her father. He used his open hand, his fist, his belt (using the end with the buckle) and occasionally an axe handle to administer his punishments beginning when she was three or four years old. Rachel's mother had done little or nothing to protect her. She was probably just as afraid of the man as Rachel.

At age fifteen, Rachel eloped with a twenty-one-year-old man from the next town. Eventually she moved to Oregon and never looked back. Her marriage was not happy, but she never gave up on it. Forty-three years later, in the summer of 1963, the phone rang in Rachel's home.

"Rachel?" asked the voice on the phone.

"Yes," she replied.

"This is your Dad."

Rachel had not seen him, spoken to him, or even received a Christmas card from him since leaving home. Now he was dying and had no one to care for him so he called his only child to ask her to return home. She made her decision, left her husband behind and returned to Kansas.

Rachel's father was in better health than she anticipated. His cancer was widespread, but grew slowly. She moved into her old room and began organizing the household. Memories from long ago hid in every corner and creaking floorboard, some returning unexpectedly. Rachel wanted to share them with her father, hoping for an apology or reconciliation. But whenever she came close to asking him about her early years and his brutal treatment, something held her back.

"I wanted to ask him about it, but every time I just got so emotional I had to leave the room," she said softly.

My next question was about her strongest emotion at those times. Was she angry with him?

"I was afraid," she replied after some thought. "I was afraid he would say it didn't happen, that he didn't beat me. I knew if he said that I couldn't stay. But how could I leave my own father to die? I couldn't face that either. So I just never brought it up even though I thought about it every day."

She hoped he might, near the end, express his regret and ask her forgiveness. Rachel spent eighteen months caring for him before he died. Even in his last lucid days, with death obviously near, he expressed no emotions toward Rachel. There was no affection, no regret, no request for forgiveness, no mention of her early years at all. There was no closure.

Rachel returned to her less than happy marriage. Within a few months, she began having difficulty with her bowels. There was constipation that would last for several days followed by an equal duration of diarrhea. She had cramps, bloating and gas pains, sometimes mild — at other times severe. She went to her doctor, who began ordering tests for infections, tumors and intestinal inflammation. All the results were normal. She tried a number of medicines. At best, they provided only temporary relief.

Rachel's illness was largely unchanged sixteen years later when her husband died in 1980. Six years after that, I saw her for the first time. She was now eighty-one and probably wondering what she was doing in yet another doctor's office. Her medical chart, still in paper form in those days, was three inches thick. We talked about her life for forty-five very sad minutes. When I got home that evening, I hugged my wife and children a little longer than usual.

Children who suffer abuse or other negative treatment learn that expressing their emotions about these events often leads to even more abuse. They learn how to control their feelings, sometimes so effectively they feel almost nothing. These buried emotions can be so strong that the mind must express them through the body if there is no other outlet. This was happening to Rachel.

Rachel's life presented her with a series of difficult choices, often between the bad and the tragic. Should she marry a man whom she did not love or remain in an abusive home? Should she stay with her husband and his economic support or try to fend for herself at a time in our history when divorced women had limited options? Should she return home to help her father or let him die alone? Rachel needed some positive options.

I recommended that she write a letter to her father, expressing her deepest thoughts and feelings about him. Obviously, since he was deceased, the letter would not be mailed, and she wasn't required to show it to anyone, unless she wanted to show it to me. To her immense credit, even though Rachel had little experience with writing, she sat down and wrote a short letter, putting feelings on a page she had shared only in talking with me. Rachel reported that her symptoms improved markedly. She said she felt relieved to "accomplish something useful" for her condition. The writing also helped her understand the many burdens she had endured and this helped her feel more positively about herself. Though I strongly recommended she see a therapist to continue the work she had started, she declined. Fortunately, Rachel's illness continued to improve even without counseling. Telling her story to me and then in more detail in the letter was enough to begin a sustained healing process. Rachel's words helped her rearrange the jigsaw pieces of her life into a new picture.

Rachel spoke easily about her difficult life. However, many patients feel they have little to say when asked to talk about themselves. In response to questions about childhood stress, I often hear "My childhood was fine."

"MY CHILDHOOD WAS FINE": DONNA

Everything in Donna's life was going extraordinarily well except for attacks of agonizing pain in the upper right corner of her abdomen that put her in the hospital twice in the last month. Donna was in her thirties and had recently experienced a number of important events: receiving her license to practice as a physician's assistant, moving to Oregon with her devoted husband, starting a job with a clinic she loved and adopting a six-month-old daughter – the couple's first child.

Donna's pain began ten years earlier when ultrasound showed gallstones. Even after surgical removal of the gallbladder, she still felt pain at times. In the months before I saw her, the pain became severe. She feared a stone had been left behind but extensive testing showed nothing wrong. What was causing the pain? Her gastroenterologist referred her to me to find out.

As is my general approach, I reviewed her life for the five major types of stress and initially turned up nothing. Donna assured me her childhood was free of stress. Donna's parents clearly wanted the best for her and always praised her when she did something well.

It was striking, however, that her symptoms worsened just at a time when she was happy with everything in her life. Her marriage, the baby, completing training, getting a good job and moving to a new state were all dreams come true for her. If Donna was a childhood stress survivor, these positive events might have contrasted strongly with her early years and created stress that I call the Good Partner/Bad Illness syndrome.

This syndrome develops in people who have experienced dysfunctional childhoods. Frequently they have had one or more difficult personal relationships during the adult years, too. Eventually, however, their self-esteem improves to the point where they can accept a much more supportive partner than they have in the past. Ironically, in the beginning these better relationships can also be stressful. Why? People not accustomed to receiving support and affection often need to make quite an adjustment when they find someone who returns their love and respect. Early in a mutually supportive relationship, attempts to be emotionally open can leave an abuse survivor feeling vulnerable or threatened. For example, some of my patients harbor a secret fear that their new partner will discover they are unworthy, especially if they reveal too much of themselves. Other patients, often those who suffered greatly as children, worry some catastrophe will occur that will end the new relationship. These anxieties sometimes can be strong enough to produce the symptoms of stress illness.

To look into Donna's childhood in more detail, I started with a remark she made during our initial interview that she was "a perfectionist." Donna had difficulty feeling satisfied no matter how carefully she did her work. This is one of the long-term consequences of childhood instability. How did she get to be that way? While Donna was growing up, her father was out of town frequently on business and not particularly interested in Donna even when he was home. She worked hard to get him to notice her achievements. Her mother often praised her, but also left Donna feeling that nothing less than her best would be good enough. As a result, she "never got into trouble," and family friends often commented on her maturity and sense of responsibility.

When Donna was ten, her family moved to France. Her mother depended on Donna for companionship during this time. If Donna tried to spend more time with her friends, her mother would express disappointment by coldly holding back attention and support. Donna's self-esteem suffered since she keenly felt her inability to meet her own needs and her mother's.

"Did anything else happen to you that might have affected your self-esteem?" I asked. Donna stood up, walked across the room and then sat on the exam table. "When I was nine, I saw a home video at my uncle's," she began. "Part of it showed me as a baby being held by my mother. My dad was there and also a little girl about six years old. I had never seen the girl before and asked my uncle who she was. He told me it was my sister Kristen."

Donna had never heard of Kristen. Donna's parents never spoke of her and there was no evidence Kristen had ever lived with them. Later Donna learned that Kristen died of cystic fibrosis at age seven. After the funeral, her parents removed everything connected to Kristen from their home. Finding out she had a sister came as a shock. "It was like finding out I was adopted," she said. "I felt devalued that my parents never told me about her."

This was a revealing example of their style of communication and emotional expression. Donna's response was to work even more diligently to be perfect so she could earn their trust and affection.

Now thirty years later, for Donna's pain to improve it was essential she understand the nature and degree of the difficulties she had overcome as a child. This was particularly difficult because her parents meant well and had done their best to care for her. I am sure part of the reason they withheld information about Kristen was that they did not want Donna to suffer any of their pain.

Donna was perceptive, insightful and verbally skilled. She was able to bring several ideas she had considered over the years into our conversation. She recalled other frustrations from her early environment. Soon Donna understood how her perfectionism developed from her struggle to prove herself to her parents. She recognized that her never-ending efforts on behalf of her job, family and friends, which left no time to care for herself, grew out of her early experiences.

When I observed that the only time she was able to think about her own needs was when she was in the hospital, Donna admitted, "Even there I brought my computer with me so I could finish some projects for work."

My advice was for her to look at everything she had accomplished and see that she deserved some regular personal time. "All I'm suggesting is that you put yourself on the list of people you take care of," I told her.

During the next few months, Donna was able to take greater satisfaction in her successes. After a lot of practice, she learned to care for herself without feeling guilty about neglecting other people. None of this happened overnight, but her pain decreased and never again became severe.

In Part II, we will meet more patients who initially reported, "My childhood was fine." When no visible illness explained their symptoms, I asked more questions and uncovered significant early issues that formed the roots of their stress illness. Also in Part II we will explore what happens when patients have trouble telling their stories or providing clues about what is underneath the surface of their symptoms. In addition, I will describe cases of multi-factored stress illness where two or more types of stress occur together. Part II stories will also illustrate how patients can take an active role in their recovery. In Part III, we will examine first how loved ones and second how the health care system can do a better job of helping the stress illness patient.

A preview of several of these issues is the following case of an adolescent stricken by both visible and stress illness that also shows how critical it is to unravel individual and family stories.

BRIAN: A SENSE OF CONTROL

Brian was a thin, exhausted eighteen-year-old whose abdominal pain had baffled six gastrointestinal specialists as he completed his tenth week in the hospital. During the previous year, two different university hospitals evaluated him without reaching a definite diagnosis. Brian's pain was getting worse with every passing month and he required an enormous amount of narcotics.

Brian enjoyed a happy life until age ten, the unfortunate year his parents divorced and he developed diabetes. Supervised by his mother, Brian did a good job taking care of the diabetes initially. In his teens, Brian's level of rebellion was no worse than most others his age, but it spilled over into using his medication less often. This allowed the diabetes to get worse, which led indirectly to an infection in his abdomen that resulted in a series of complications. Just when it seemed these problems were finally over, Brian began to complain of abdominal pain again. At first, it would come and go, but after a while it was present more often than not. Initially mild, the pain became more severe at times. Diagnostic tests were inconclusive.

Soon after Brian turned eighteen, he returned to the hospital because his pain was out of control. His doctors ordered more blood tests, x-rays, CAT scans, ultrasound exams and nuclear medicine studies. He had some abnormal blood tests related to diabetes but nothing to explain his pain. Soon his narcotic dose reached amounts usually given to patients with severe pain from widespread cancer (which he definitely did not have). Brian's pain was relieved temporarily after each increase in dosage, but it was never long before he was asking for more.

After ten weeks in the hospital, Brian's mother Janet had seen enough. Janet had been by Brian's side throughout the ordeal and could not tolerate seeing her son in pain any longer. She told the nurse it was intolerable and unethical for her son's pain not to be controlled. Janet had seen a brochure about the hospital's Ethics Service some weeks earlier and asked for a consultation. I am the Ethics Director for our medical group and I happened to be on call for this service that day.

I had seen Brian briefly during his first month in the hospital, but did not know him well. In reviewing his records, the extensive evaluation showed only a few abnormalities, none of which could account for such severe pain.

I asked him in detail about stresses in each of the five categories (present day, childhood, trauma, depression, anxiety). His parent's divorce, the diabetes and the many medical complications had certainly taken their toll. But Brian revealed nothing capable of putting a young man into a hospital on round-the-clock narcotics.

When I look for stress in an adolescent, I am especially interested in learning about problems in the family. As I listen to the patient, I keep in mind that it is common for teens to report only a fraction of the true level of difficulty they are experiencing. This is, in part, because of their strong desire to meet parental and family expectations. Since information from the teen patient might be incomplete, it is often necessary to interview more than one family member to understand a family's stresses. This is helpful not only in diagnosis, but also, later on, to help the family interact in a new way. Changing a parent's behavior is sometimes the best way to relieve an adolescent's illness.

Brian mentioned a few times that his mother might be too concerned about his care. I remembered seeing Janet almost every time I walked by Brian's hospital room. The hospital chapel, empty on a Wednesday morning, was the only quiet place I could find for Janet and me to talk. She was gracious and appreciated my involvement. We began with the idea that getting to know other family members might lead to help for Brian. Janet was quite willing to tell me about herself.

Janet's father was a busy executive who worked long hours and had little time or energy for his family. Janet's mother might have been manic-depressive, suffered for years from pain of uncertain cause, frequently drank too much alcohol, rarely expressed affection for anyone, was often manipulative, and occasionally spent time in the hospital or a psychiatric facility.

Janet's mother also used narcotics for her pain and Janet was heavily involved in providing care for her mother from a young age. At times, this even included giving her mother injections. As a girl, Janet's only real hope for getting support or affection came from taking on responsibilities far beyond her years. Janet admitted to suffering from emotional problems as a teenager, but recovered after a few years without professional intervention.

After the diagnosis of Brian's diabetes, Janet was once again a caregiver. Instantly she was back in the role she knew so well. She took full responsibility for managing all aspects of her son's care and other aspects of his life if they might affect his health.

Now I could better understand Brian's inner anguish. Brian recognized that when he was younger, it was essential to his health to have support from Janet. However, at age eighteen, Brian felt he had no more control over his life than he had at age ten. Caught between his illness, his doctors and his mother, Brian led a life that was so restricted there was a part of him that wanted to scream. Actually, he was screaming, but inside — where it took the form of abdominal pain.

Janet was quite perceptive about these issues. She was also willing to do anything to help her son. We agreed she would continue to provide emotional support, but Brian would now make all the decisions about his health care and, within broad limits, his life in general. Janet and I walked back to her son's room and shared the results of our discussion with Brian.

This was asking a lot from both of them. I was asking Janet to give up a role she had fulfilled successfully for most of her life. I was asking Brian to take on a huge new responsibility. It was not at all clear that Janet could manage it, that Brian could cope with it or that the pain would respond to it. Still, since all the medical approaches had failed, there was not much to lose by trying.

One week later, Brian was able to leave the hospital with just tablets for pain. One month later, the pain was gone and the narcotics stopped. Brian took to his new freedom and power like a fledgling out of its nest. His mother rose to the occasion magnificently, changed her old behavior patterns, and watched with great pride as her son became an adult.

Brian's new sense of control over his life was a cornerstone to his healing. The opened eyes and opened minds that he and his mother were willing to have about themselves and each other were essential to this achievement.

A NEW AWARENESS

As we continue, I hope that a new awareness is dawning within you, perhaps opening your eyes and mind about who you are, how your past and present connect and how stress might or might not be impacting you.

In Part II, several stories illustrate each of the five types of stress. You will learn that it is possible to prevail over the most difficult conditions, partly because the challenges ahead are usually smaller than those you have already overcome. My patients have taught me they have a light inside that can reveal not only previously invisible problems, but also the path that leads beyond them.

PART II
CAUSES, CONSEQUENCES, AND TREATMENT OF STRESS ILLNESS

We shall not cease from exploration
And the end of all our exploring
Will be to arrive where we started
And know the place for the first time.

– T.S. Eliot

CHAPTER 3
CHILDHOOD STRESS

Stress won't go away if an unresolved conflict exists.
It's like painting primer over rotting wood.

– Scott Morton

CHILDHOOD STRESS: KAREN

WHEN KAREN'S DIARRHEA CAUSED HER TO LOSE NINETY POUNDS IN EIGHTEEN months, you did not need to be a doctor to see she had a serious problem. She was afraid she had cancer, but looked surprisingly healthy at 115 pounds. Her physician hospitalized her for tests, all of which were normal. As we talked, she mentioned a remarkable feature of her illness: she had severe diarrhea only three or four days each week. The other days she felt fine. Few if any diseases caused by tumors, inflammation, infection or other visible abnormality would cause diarrhea that fluctuated so dramatically.

Stress illness, on the other hand, is often associated with highly variable symptoms, but none of her other doctors had inquired about stress. Our conversation reviewed all five types. Karen was thirty-four and married to a bus driver, and they had a two-year-old son. She enjoyed her job making baked goods for a supermarket. She had never suffered a significant trauma and had no symptoms of anxiety or depression. Karen also had not experienced any obvious form of childhood mistreatment. If her illness was due to stress, I was missing something. My inquiry about childhood stress had focused on specific issues such as molestation and parental alcohol abuse. Perhaps I had been too specific. I tried to think of a more general and open-ended question.

"Did anything happen to you as a child that significantly lowered your self-esteem?" I asked.

"Oh, yes!" she replied immediately. "Every night at dinner my mom would talk to my brother and me about everything we had done wrong that day and what we should do to improve."

Night after night as she grew up, she endured this criticism. There was far less in the way of praise or support and Karen's self esteem suffered significantly. Interviews with thousands of survivors of child abuse have taught me the enduring power of Karen's experience. Children will go through walls to please a parent and only a few stop trying when they become adults.

"How is your relationship with her now?" I asked.

"She's still doing it," she sighed.

Six months after Karen's son was born her mother started finding fault with her again. Not only did she criticize Karen's skills as a mother, but she commented on the shortcomings of her infant son, too. Karen's mother was important to her and she wanted her to have contact with her grandchild, but at the same time, she was very unhappy about her unrelenting disapproval. Sometimes Karen did not know if she wanted to hug her mother or kick her off the front porch. Karen definitely did not want her son to suffer as she had. There seemed to be no way out. The diarrhea began, her appetite declined and she shed five pounds each month.

"Karen, after all that you've been through, it's no wonder you became ill," I said.

As we spoke in her hospital room, she began to understand the impact of her mother's behavior on her self-esteem. After a long discussion, Karen understood how the return of her critical words left her feelings for her mother trapped between affection and resentment. She recognized how single-minded she had become in her endless attempts to gain her mother's approval. She became confident that she could share her concerns with her mother. I saw Karen's shoulders relax. Then she leaned back in the bed and took a deep breath. It was rewarding to see her determined expression as she spoke about her plans for coping with her mother.

The next day she was able to leave the hospital and the diarrhea never returned. She regained fifteen pounds in three weeks and kept her weight steady thereafter. Then Karen and her mother had a conversation that helped clarify the harm of her mother's well-intentioned comments. The mother was defensive at first, but eventually she understood Karen's point of view. Their interactions became much more positive.

Karen's case illustrates the central importance of self-esteem. She never suffered any form of abuse that involved physical contact and her childhood home was stable, yet her mother's damaging words lowered Karen's self-esteem as much as other forms of abuse could have. To some people her mother's criticism and the prospect of enduring it for years to come might not seem sufficient to cause a severe illness. However, children will do nearly anything to earn parental approval. When they receive no praise, when nothing they accomplish is good enough, this emotional abuse can cause enduring harm that has led to physical illness in scores of my patients.

The repetition of Karen's childhood stress in her adult years is one way these issues can cause symptoms. In many other patients, the connection between adverse early experience and stress illness later in life is not obvious. A large number of my patients become ill years or even decades after they have grown and moved away from their dysfunctional family. In these cases, the illness is the result of the long-term consequences of childhood stress, a process usually hidden from those experiencing it. You will learn about this process in the next three sections and then more illustrative stories follow.

CHILDHOOD STRESS CONSEQUENCES: EARLY STAGES

The emotional pain of childhood stress can endure for a lifetime and is a common cause of stress illness. Illness can begin during childhood, during adolescence or soon after a young adult leaves home. In other patients, illness might not emerge until much later in adult life after a long and complex process that begins with damage to the child's self-esteem. Review of this process begins in this section and continues in the two sections that follow. Understanding the steps involved is essential to overcoming the illness.

Many people assume that damage to a child's self-esteem comes only from physical or sexual abuse. However, Karen's story in the last section shows that other forms of childhood stress can be just as harmful. Here is a list of problems that can lower a child's self-esteem:

- Abuse (Emotional, Verbal, Physical, Sexual)
- Alcohol or drug abuse in the home
- Violence in the home
- Standards for parental approval that are too high
- Neglect or abandonment
- Negative treatment by peers
- Having to take on parental or adult responsibilities when too young

Many patients believe their childhood experiences could not be responsible for illness because others have experienced far worse and do not appear to be ill. My response is to point out that any of the stresses on the list above are capable of causing illness, that everyone reacts to stress in their own way, and that most of my patients have endured far more than they realize at first.

How did my patients respond to difficulties when they were children? They had limited options for coping. To survive emotionally and physically, many of them worked hard to please the authority figures, care for the family and keep disruptions to a minimum. Many helped raise their siblings, cleaned the home, paid bills, shopped for food and clothing and did the laundry. They often worked just as diligently at school or in extracurricular activities.

They also learned to be aware of small details that might tip them off to a problem. This is because, for many of these children, their home resembled a minefield. They could never be sure when the next physical or emotional blow was going to come. Was there alcohol on Dad's breath? Did Mom just bang the frying pan on the stove? The home demanded constant vigilance.

Children who learn these skills usually continue to use them as adults. They work hard and are reliable, detail-oriented and able to get things done. Since they are personally familiar with human suffering, they also tend to be compassionate. Childhood stress survivors often become people you would wish to have as your marriage partner, co-worker, supervisor, employee, friend or neighbor. At times, however, the survivor's fine qualities might go too far and cause them stress. The meticulous worker could become a perpetually unsatisfied perfectionist. Caring individuals might look to the needs of everyone else, but never get around to nurturing themselves.

Surviving a dysfunctional home can also cause people to have a number of other significant problems including:

- Long-term relationships with partners who mistreat them. People accustomed to poor treatment might find it natural to form relationships with people who are disrespectful, who attempt to control them or who subject them to verbal or physical violence. These "bad partners" occur frequently in the early adult lives of childhood stress survivors.
- Addiction(s) to nicotine, alcohol, drugs, food, sex, work, gambling, shopping or exercise. Many people develop addictive behavior because it can provide some relief from the emotional consequences of a difficult childhood.
- A quick temper or a tendency toward violence. Children in dysfunctional homes learn to suppress their anger. They continue to do so as adults, but some of them live just below the boiling point. Relatively small events might trigger an outburst.
- Abusing their own children or fear that they will abuse them.
- Anorexia nervosa, an eating disorder where patients maintain a body weight low enough to be unhealthy or even life threatening. Additional issues include fear of gaining weight, fear of becoming fat (even when quite thin) and distortion of the body image so that there is no concern about being seriously underweight. For some people with this condition, controlling their weight could provide a form of relief when everything else feels chaotic.
- Bulimia, another eating disorder common in survivors of childhood stress. Bulimics suffer repeated episodes of binge eating (consuming large quantities in a short period, often with a sense that the eating is not controllable). Associated with this might be attempts to reduce the caloric load of the eating by such means as inducing vomiting, use of laxatives or enemas or heavy exercise.

- Mental health problems such as "nervous breakdowns" or suicide attempts.
- Inability to sense or verbalize their own feelings. When there are few safe outlets for self-expression, children learn how to control their emotions so well they have difficulty feeling them.
- Self-mutilation. Some individuals reach a point where they feel almost no emotion, which is a very unpleasant state. Acts of self-mutilation such as cutting or burning can provide a way to feel something and can serve as a distraction from emotional pain. For some, self-mutilation is also an act of self-punishment that alleviates guilt for assumed "bad" behavior. This "bad" behavior might be "allowing" someone to abuse the person sexually.
- Unhealthy behaviors including overeating, smoking and lack of exercise.
- Increased risk of becoming a victim of assault, rape or domestic violence.
- Poor self-esteem, feeling ashamed of past events.

These personal problems sometimes are significant enough to cause stress illness. Many of these issues can also cause dysfunctional home survivors to feel ashamed of themselves, which compounds the stress. Some relief from shame comes from recognizing that many of these problems result from a mind under pressure doing whatever is necessary to survive. For example, some individuals might become obese to protect themselves from unwanted sexual attention. Others might slip into anorexia to find a measure of control when all else feels chaotic. Drug use and other addictions can alleviate emotional pain. Feeling the wounds of self-mutilation can give the relief and distraction of having a sensation when there are few other feelings available.

Taking personal responsibility for overcoming the problems listed above is clearly essential. The next step is recognizing that these issues are common consequences of dysfunctional environments. The journey to recovery begins when pride in having survived replaces shame and regret.

As you can see, childhood stress survivors tend to have a blend of positive and negative personal characteristics. Fortunately, in most of my patients, the good qualities endure and the bad ones diminish. This is because the survivors' personal strength, energy, compassion and dedication produce strong approval and support from the world outside the family. This reinforces positive traits and helps overcome weaknesses. Over time (sometimes a long time), the good feedback and a human being's natural ability to recover from adversity leads to steady improvement in self-esteem.

Siri is an excellent example. For nearly three years, she had pains in her lower abdomen that occurred on the left side some days, on the right other days, deep in the pelvis at times and in her low back at still other times. Born in rural Thailand, her father verbally abused her almost daily, leaving her self-esteem in a deep hole. She moved to Bangkok as a young woman. There Siri found success working as a computer programmer, playing with a musical quartet and earning extra money as a fashion model. Her personal life did not work out so well though, since her first husband slept with other women and often slapped her. She experienced abdominal pain during the marriage that was relieved soon after their divorce.

A few years later, Siri met her current husband on an internet site for American men interested in marrying Thai women. Unfortunately, this marriage was not much better than her first. He appeared not to appreciate her beauty and talent. He belittled her for errors in speaking English. He insisted she avoid talking to other men unless he was present. He deposited her paychecks in his bank account, limited her personal spending money and strictly controlled how she spent her free time. Her abdominal pains soon returned. I never met her husband but I could not imagine how anyone could be so blind to her beauty, intelligence and kindness.

At first, Siri had been grateful that her American husband did not hit her and she tried to adapt herself to his needs. However, her self-esteem began to respond to her tremendous popularity at the small software firm where she worked. After a while she began to hope that one day her husband would stop being so disrespectful. The idea that she deserved a husband who loved her at least as much as her co-workers did was still in her future.

I asked about her performance ratings at work. "Always an A," she replied.

Then I asked her to estimate the performance rating her husband would give. She smiled ruefully and said, "Always a D." I asked her to consider which of these evaluations was closer to the truth.

"After everything you have overcome in your life, I would certainly give you an A," I assured her. I also pointed out that her abdominal pains had occurred twice in her life, both in association with disrespectful husbands.

Siri's self-esteem was steadily approaching the level it would have reached long ago if not for her father and husbands. Soon she would have a new attitude about herself and would no longer tolerate her husband's lack of respect. This is the next step in the process of recovery from childhood stress. An acronym captures the essence of the new attitude: it is what I call I.D.B., which stands for "I Deserve Better." You might recall the story of Catherine who survived childhood molestation but became ill thirty years later. Her symptoms began when she reached the "I Deserve Better" stage and quit working for her "total jerk" boss.

CHILDHOOD STRESS CONSEQUENCES: I DESERVE BETTER

Positive experiences in the adult world help childhood stress survivors learn they deserve better than past or present mistreatment. Self-esteem builds steadily and eventually survivors accept that they deserve as much respect as anyone else. Once this happens, there is no turning back. This new attitude results in a re-evaluation of one's life and everyone in it. This is crucial in overcoming the effects of a dysfunctional childhood. Yet this process also can be so difficult that stress illness results.

Why is this stage so hard? First, people become less tolerant of disrespectful treatment. They might insist on changes in behavior from their spouse, parents, children and co-workers and this is rarely easy to accomplish. Some find they must end a difficult marital or working relationship.

Second, new personal relationships can form. These can be much more mutually supportive than relationships experienced in the past but, as we saw in the story about Donna, the "Good Partner/Bad Illness" syndrome can be the result. This is what happened to Martha.

I learned about Martha's Good Partner/Bad Illness syndrome almost by accident. Her self-esteem was low as a child because both parents were alcoholics, but now, at age thirty-seven, her life was going well. Her self-esteem had improved to the point where she could accept a positive, mutually supportive relationship with her fiancé Ron. Then she suddenly developed severe constipation the preceding April. We met in October after six months of diagnostic tests (with no evaluation for stress) had failed to detect a cause. As I examined her, I commented on the glittering diamond on her left hand. "Ron likes to do everything in a big way," she responded. "We got engaged last April." Since her illness also started in April, I pinned her down on exact dates and learned that her bowel trouble started a few days after she accepted Ron's proposal. "You don't think they're related, do you?" she asked.

I was not sure so I asked her to tell me more about Ron. There was no question that Martha loved him, that he was by far the most caring person ever in her life and that she wanted very much to marry him. Unfortunately, because her previous relationships with men had been disastrous, she could not help being a little afraid about similar problems occurring in the future with Ron. In addition, Martha's self-esteem was still so low she was afraid Ron might someday decide she was not who he wanted. She admitted there was no justification for these fears, but they remained quite real to her. Using the treatment techniques described later in this book and with the help of a therapist, Martha's concerns about Ron diminished steadily. By their wedding day, she no longer had a problem with constipation.

Meeting a good partner is not the only type of positive experience that can trigger stress illness. One of my patients became ill on receiving her Ph.D. after many years of sacrifice and hard work. The contrast between this achievement and her low self-esteem from childhood was difficult for her to reconcile. Another patient became ill soon after receiving the Person of the Year award from four hundred fellow employees. His mother had treated him poorly as a child and the award made him recognize that his mother and his co-workers could not both be right about him.

Stress from a good partner or life-affirming event is only temporary. The long-term benefits far outweigh the short-term adjustments and support from the partner or pride in the accomplishment builds self-acceptance. Consequently, stress from adapting to the new circumstances does not last long.

The change to an I.D.B. attitude also changes perceptions about childhood experiences. I.D.B. can also stand for I Deserved Better. When a person decides they deserve as much respect as anyone else, they might correctly conclude they deserved respect as children also. Resentment and anger about their mistreatment begin to grow, often without conscious awareness. Whether an individual is aware of the emotion or not, the anger is real and powerful.

CHILDHOOD STRESS CONSEQUENCES: ANGER

Anger about childhood mistreatment is an unpleasant emotion, so people often suppress it consciously or unconsciously. Another reason for the suppression occurs when individuals who mistreated the patient are not able to receive or respond to the anger. They might be deceased, have no known address or be mentally or physically incompetent. They might also be unwilling or emotionally unable to respond to a discussion of the past.

Another reason for suppressing anger is a desire for reconciliation. Few of my patients ever completely lose hope that their family will one day recognize the harm that occurred. Often my patients fear that hope will be lost if they vent anger at a parent.

Finally, for many, survival of a difficult childhood depended on controlling emotions. In dysfunctional homes, there is often little tolerance for emotional expression by children. Some children learn to control their feelings so well they become less and less aware of them. They just do not feel those emotions any more.

For all these reasons, many of my patients don't recognize how much anger is locked inside them and consequently their emotions can't be expressed easily in words. Under these circumstances, where can this anger go? Some people release it onto people or objects around them. They raise their voice, lose their temper, hit people, destroy things or might be prone to "road rage." In many others, the stress response center sends anger into the body and stress illness is the result. Sasha had this problem.

Sasha was in her forties and had suffered episodes of severe gagging for about three years. These attacks went on for up to ten minutes and occurred several times each month. Gagging often started when she had something in her mouth like a toothbrush, cigarette or food. At other times, there was no obvious common factor. One curious statement she made was about feeling angry while her attacks were occurring. Initially, I assumed this anger came from frustration with the symptoms, but that proved to be a superficial interpretation.

All Sasha's tests were normal. She had no major current life stresses, no traumas, no symptoms of depression or anxiety and she loved her job as a substitute teacher. Initially she described her childhood as free of significant problems, that it was "fine, nothing bad." However, Sasha had many of the personal qualities and life experiences discussed in the section on long-term consequences of childhood stress. Her self-esteem was poor, she had divorced three times and she would not even consider quitting smoking.

Therefore, I was suspicious that something had happened to her as a child. I asked her if she could think of anything about her childhood that made her angry. She replied, "I remember one time my father pushed my mother into the refrigerator during an argument."

When I asked her if fights like that happened very often, she told me they occurred several times each month. My next question was to ask if Sasha's father had ever fought with her.

"Yes, he used to say I was worthless." Tears appeared in her eyes as she said this. "Also, he never was home for my birthday." It turned out her birthday was on the first day of hunting season. For some reason he couldn't wait until the second day.

Next I wondered if Sasha's father had ever hit, punched, slapped, or kicked her. She admitted that he had but then added "not as much as with my mom. And it didn't really bother me."

As a young doctor, I was often surprised to hear stories like this coming from people who, five minutes earlier, had told me their childhood was "fine." These revelations do not surprise me nearly as much today.

"Was there ever any form of sexual abuse from your father or anyone else?" Many of my patients are shocked when I ask this question, but Sasha looked like she was ready to tell me the answer even before I asked.

"The day before my sixteenth birthday he fondled my breasts. He had never done anything like that before. The next day he went hunting again like nothing had happened."

"Was that the only time?"

"After that first time he started doing it over and over. Then when I was seventeen, he reached under my skirt. That was when I moved out."

Sasha lived with the family of a friend until she graduated from high school. Then she got a job and an apartment and avoided her parents as much as possible. After she finished describing these problems, she said again, they "didn't bother me."

But it turned out that three years earlier, just at the time when her gagging episodes began, Sasha's father, now in his late sixties, developed a chronic illness and needed her help. After avoiding him for most of her adult life, she suddenly found herself in contact with him four or five days each week. Despite his illness and dependence on Sasha, he often belittled her as he had done when she was a girl. Part of Sasha became justifiably outraged, but she suppressed these emotions so well she truly believed she was not angry and the child abuse had not affected her. Her stress response center sent the rage into the back of her throat and the gagging was the result.

Our review of the negative events in Sasha's childhood started her thinking about them again. Soon she realized these issues had been troubling her for many years. I recommended Sasha write about these early events and this helped her get in touch with the locked up emotions. The more the emotions spilled out onto the page, the less power they had to produce symptoms. The gagging attacks began to fade away. She started seeing a counselor and before long, she was able to confront her father and insist he treat her with respect. The gagging attacks stopped completely after that.

Rage channeled into the body, as in Sasha's case, is a common cause of stress illness. Treatment starts with identifying the source(s) of the anger followed by re-directing these feelings into written or spoken words. In addition to releasing emotions, the writing helped Sasha comprehend the severity of the problems she had overcome. Eventually she was able to think of her childhood as a challenge she had triumphed over rather than as a source of humiliation.

Now that you understand the long-term consequences of childhood stress, the following stories will further illustrate the range of problems that can result.

CHILDHOOD STRESS: WENDY

Dr. Jim Burns is an old friend and his patients like him as much as I do. Except for Wendy. When Jim called to ask me to see Wendy as soon as possible, he warned me that she was calling our medical director every week to complain about her health care in general and him in particular. Three other doctors had treated Wendy in the last year and she had "fired" them all for not finding the cause of her illness.

Wendy was forty-nine and earned her living selling a line of cosmetics in women's homes. Her symptoms consisted of severe pain along the right side of her body from her shoulder to her upper thigh. At times, she also had vomiting, diarrhea or both. She had spent a total of nearly two months in the hospital during eight separate admissions. Examination by several specialists and two psychiatrists found no explanation for her problems. She was convinced she had cancer.

I was expecting to meet an angry woman, but fortunately she seemed willing to give me a chance. We began to review the five types of stress, finding Wendy had several symptoms of depression. However, her depression did not seem severe enough to produce such a debilitating illness by itself.

Wendy's childhood history contained a shock. "When I was five years old, my parents went on a trip to Montana, leaving me and my younger sister with the neighbors," she began. "Three days later they called and said they were getting a divorce and would not be coming back." This was the last Wendy saw of her parents for the next twenty years. A succession of relatives took on Wendy and her sister like unwanted baggage. Wendy dedicated herself to taking care of her sister as best she could. Her self-esteem, not surprisingly, was abysmal.

At age seventeen, Wendy married a man who abused her physically and verbally. After he raped her at knifepoint when she was twenty-eight, she left him. Soon after, Wendy married her current husband. He was an alcoholic, but not violent and "he's been drinking a little less the last few years."

After fifteen years working in low-paying service jobs and about five months before her illness began, Wendy began selling cosmetics and the appalling story of her life finally took a positive turn. She proved to be quite talented at the cosmetics business. In a short time, she was able to quit her job at a photocopy shop and soon began making far more money than she ever had before. Wendy's fast start earned her a great deal of respect at the cosmetics company. Soon she began to respect herself and, consequently, Wendy became less tolerant of her husband's shortcomings. She stopped trying to meet his every need the way she had for her first husband and (as a child) for her sister and her relatives. Then the pain, vomiting episodes and diarrhea began.

With her success in business, Wendy reached the "I Deserve Better" stage of her recovery from a traumatic childhood. She became convinced that she deserved respect from everyone in her life. When she talked about her parents, she was calm and outwardly unemotional. However, the words she spoke revealed how much she "hated" them for leaving, how "mad" she was that they had never apologized and how "terrible" it had been for her little sister. Though the words revealed her emotions, her manner and tone concealed them. No one, not even Wendy herself, was aware of the amount of anger concealed inside because she expressed rage through her body instead of in words or actions. Her painful symptoms were the result.

Although two psychiatrists had failed to find her problem, Wendy agreed to talk to a new therapist about the issues we had uncovered. At my suggestion, she began writing a letter to her parents that she later described as "the hardest thing I've ever done." She also agreed to take an antidepressant medication that helped her sleeping and fatigue considerably. Wendy's pain and digestive symptoms vanished completely in less than ten days, which was much sooner than I expected. She continued to work with the therapist for over a year and her business became even more successful.

CHILDHOOD STRESS: EMMA

Just looking at Emma's massive medical record discouraged me. She suffered from bowel problems for nearly *eight decades* with no obvious benefit from any of her encounters with the medical profession. Emma was eighty-eight years old with loosely curled snow-white hair. She answered questions thoughtfully and in detail. Her eyes searched my face to see if I had the solution to her abdominal cramps and alternating diarrhea and constipation. These symptoms were not severe; sometimes they even went away, but never for more than a week or two. None of her scores of diagnostic tests had ever revealed an abnormality and no treatment worked for long.

Emma was not depressed or anxious. Her life was lonely at times (her husband had died many years ago), but was hardly stressful. Her symptoms began when she was a child. "Was there any trouble in your life when you were young?" I asked.

Emma grew up on a farm in a valley within the Rocky Mountains. Her parents loved each other, their two sons and three daughters. There was no abuse, no alcoholism, and no pressure. In many ways, it was a storybook place. Emma was the oldest daughter. When she was six years old, another boy was born. With the large number of other children and the work of the farm, the mother relied on Emma to care for the baby. Emma took to this task as she would to a favorite doll. She held, fed, dressed, changed, played with, sang to and slept with her brother. They were inseparable.

Two years later the infant developed a fever. Medical resources in rural areas in 1918 were not abundant. By the time the doctor diagnosed appendicitis, it was too late and he died.

Emma went into shock. Her ability to express emotions shut down temporarily. At the funeral, an aunt pointed out she was the only person in the church who was not crying. Her tone implied that Emma must not care about her brother's death. Her guilt, already intense, went off the scale. In telling this story, her eyes watered. Her rapid flowing speech slowed to a trickle and her lively face softened. She looked away and into the landscape painting on the exam room wall.

Not surprisingly, her brother's death affected her entire life. Within two months, she began caring for a newborn on a neighboring farm. Sometimes, though, she could not make the walk to the neighbors because her stomach had started to bother her. The pains persisted during high school and college where she supported herself by caring for children. Emma chose pediatric nursing for her career. She married and had several children of her own, raising them carefully to adulthood. Through all these years her symptoms persisted.

She stopped talking and looked at the landscape painting again. After a while she turned back and said, "You know, you're the first doctor that ever asked me about my brother. What do you think I should do?"

What could I recommend that would alleviate eighty years of guilt? Many of my patients who struggle for personal insight have understood themselves more clearly by imagining another person coping with the same problems. I recommended that Emma walk by an elementary school at recess so she could see the children on the playground. I told her to pick out a girl who reminded her of herself at age eight. While watching this young girl, I asked Emma to imagine what a child could do to save a two-year-old with a ruptured appendix in the days before antibiotics. Once she had done that, I suggested she return home and write a letter to the infant brother, asking forgiveness. She thanked me quietly and did not see a physician about her illness for several years.

I was surprised three years later when she returned to my office with similar symptoms. She insisted on more testing and when this was again normal, I asked her if she wrote the letter to her brother. She seemed surprised by the question. Not only had she not written the letter, she also didn't recall this recommendation or much of the conversation leading up to it.

I wondered what happened since our first encounter. Was her memory poor and had she simply forgotten our discussion? This did not seem likely since she lived alone, managed her affairs competently and remembered many other details without difficulty. Was it simply that there was no link between her brother's death and her illness? This was possible, though the coincidence between the death and the start of the symptoms was difficult to set aside. In addition, without any special treatment, she had felt better for several years after our first visit. I wondered if our discussion had been so emotional for her that she was unable to listen to my recommendations. Or perhaps eighty years was simply too much time for her to reach back and release buried emotions.

Stress illness treatment is often subject to uncertainty and Emma is a good example. Confirmation of the diagnosis comes only when the symptoms stop. Even when I am confident that I have identified the major stresses responsible for an illness, the patient might not be able to make use of this information and cope with the problem right away. Patience, encouragement, counseling, persistence and judicious use of medical tests are all part of the process that leads to progress.

Emma and I reviewed some of the key ideas from our first visit. I asked Emma what she thought about these. She was not sure, but admitted, "You might be right" and said she would "think about" writing the letter to her brother. Since then she has again had few medical visits for this problem.

CHILDHOOD STRESS: DAN

Dan's medical chart was over three inches thick. He was fifty-nine and had suffered chest and neck pain since he was nineteen. In those forty years, there had been no definite diagnosis and no successful treatment. He was also a challenge to interview. His answers would have been a credit to a mafia boss on the witness stand. He gave almost nothing away, saying only several dozen words in thirty minutes.

Fortunately, his wife Julia was more than willing to share his story, especially when I asked about his childhood.

"His father used to beat him," she said.

"How often did that happen?" I asked.

Julia glanced at Dan for permission to go on. Dan did not move. "He would hit him all the time," Julia continued. "And not just with his fists. He used sticks, belts, two-by-fours, anything."

"Whatever he could get his hands on," Dan added.

I remember thinking how tragic it was that none of his doctors had asked him about his childhood during decades of normal diagnostic tests and unsuccessful treatments. I let Julia continue the story.

"When he was sixteen he couldn't take it any longer," she said. He dropped out of school, left home and went to work in the woods. "He never saw his father again." Four years after leaving home the pains began and they had bothered him more often than not ever since.

We spoke about the ability of stress, even from long ago, to cause physical pain. We talked about how commonly this occurs when verbal outlets for anger are not available. He listened carefully, nodded a few times, but said nothing. I recommended he attend a course for Adult Children of Dysfunctional Families, consisting of a two-hour class every week for eight weeks.

Dan looked skeptical but Julia was all for it. "I'll make sure he goes," she said.

They returned for Dan's follow-up visit after taking the course. This time Dan told the story. By the second week of the course, he had said nothing to his classmates. Then he surprised himself by sharing a little about his childhood abuse. After the first two sentences, he stopped, suddenly realizing that a dozen strangers now knew what he had shared only with Julia and me. It must have seemed to the class he had more to say because no one spoke.

"I kept waiting for someone else to say something, but no one did," he said. "So finally I just started talking again."

His third sentence came out, followed by a fourth, and then everything boiling within him for all those decades burst out. He spoke non-stop for over half an hour and went home that night not sure what had happened. In the weeks that followed, the supportive attention of his classmates and the opportunity to hear their stories of adversity began to change how Dan thought about himself. He recognized that he was not alone in his suffering. As he encouraged his classmates to take pride in what they had overcome, he realized he was speaking to himself as well.

One day as he drove to class, he realized he had not experienced any pains for over three weeks. A month later during our follow-up visit, the pain still had not returned. Not only has he remained well ever since, but now when there is something on his mind, he speaks up for himself.

"MY CHILDHOOD WAS FINE": KEVIN

Many patients with stress illness had no adverse experiences in childhood. Other patients, like Donna, who learned about her dead sister from a videotape, do not perceive how much difficulty they overcame as a child. "My childhood was fine," they say, but further questioning reveals significant problems. As children, they suppressed their emotions to such a degree that as adults they do not recall their experience as difficult.

In other patients who tell me they had no childhood troubles, the stresses were present, but they were subtle. During an interview, my suspicion about childhood issues increases when a person's life history indicates they had low self-esteem in the past. Kevin is one example.

He was a middle-aged, recently remarried, articulate executive at a small but successful advertising agency. Ten months earlier, he had experienced an excruciating episode of pain in the liver area that doubled him over. Kevin's worried wife rushed him to the hospital where none of the diagnostic tests showed the slightest problem. He received narcotics for the pain and by the time they wore off, the pain was gone and he returned home.

He felt well for three months, but then another attack occurred. He returned to the emergency room where his experience was the same as during the first episode. Four months later, another attack occurred followed by two more at shorter intervals. More tests had the same normal results.

Kevin was not in pain when I met him and was easygoing and friendly. He gave detailed answers to all my questions and accepted the idea that stress was one possible explanation for his pain. He had no symptoms of depression or anxiety, nor were there any traumatic events in his life. He was busy at work, but was careful to preserve time for himself and his wife. He had been married to Jo for just over a year and described her as low-key and supportive. They were clearly devoted to each other. As a child, Kevin had not suffered any abuse nor had there been any violence, alcoholism or drug abuse in his home.

After questioning Kevin for over half an hour, I could find no reason for him to have stress illness. Since all the appropriate diagnostic tests were normal, I had difficulty thinking of a way to help him. I asked about his life during his twenties hoping to learn something useful. Fortunately, several clues jumped out. Kevin's first wife had been verbally abusive, drank too much alcohol, smoked a lot of marijuana and failed to provide any emotional support as he made a series of difficult career choices. He stayed with this woman for nearly a decade because he "wanted to avoid getting divorced like my parents did." Kevin's ex-wife sounded much like the "bad partner" that is so common in the early lives of survivors of childhood stress.

Kevin also had not mentioned his parents' divorce in describing his "stress-free" childhood. Kevin's parents divorced during his teen years, which was a significant emotional blow. He developed a drug habit soon afterwards, which continued until his mid-twenties. Kevin admitted his low self-esteem as a teen and during his first marriage persisted until several years after his divorce, despite success in the workplace.

By the time he met Jo his self-esteem was much better. When Jo told him he was wonderful, he believed her. Yet, Kevin's abdominal pain began soon after they were married. It seemed possible he had the "Good Partner/Bad Illness" syndrome described in the last chapter. Recall that this occurs when the support of a new and good partner leads to resentment about earlier poor treatment. Sometimes the growing resentment has no outlet except the body and illness results.

The events of Kevin's twenties and thirties reminded me of the life histories of my patients whose self-esteem suffered when they were children. His parents' divorce had been emotionally difficult, but did not seem enough by itself to explain the drug abuse that followed or his abdominal pain now. It seemed likely he had more stress as a child than he appreciated at the time and I shared this concern with him. Kevin thought for a few moments and then provided the solution to his mysterious illness.

"There were five of us kids and when we were growing up, we all had to compete with each other for praise," he said. The children were all distinguished in their academic and social abilities. Their peers and teachers thought highly of them. However, to win praise at home, they had to be better than their brothers and sisters. Kevin remembered that he and a sister had once "wished they were dumb" so there would be no need to compete with the other siblings.

Kevin had persuaded himself that the family competition was reasonable. After all, Kevin thought, "How else could you tell if you were doing well?" except by competing. But the competition never let up. Kevin's childhood was a constant battle to outshine his siblings and earn his parents' attention. Unfortunately, his parents praised their children so infrequently and the effort needed to earn approval was so great that Kevin's self-esteem settled at a far lower level than his accomplishments warranted, making him even more vulnerable when schoolmates teased him about his weight (he was heavy in high school). His parents' divorce pushed him even lower. The low self-esteem also helped explain why he married his first wife, who treated him so poorly: that relationship was consistent with what he had endured as a child.

Kevin was not convinced that any of this was relevant to his illness. It was his perception that his childhood experience was not especially harsh. I looked for a better way to understand how much pressure Kevin had experienced as a boy. He had mentioned during our discussion that his best friend Clay had a delightful six-year-old daughter named Victoria. I asked Kevin if he would be comfortable making Victoria compete for praise. He became quiet for a moment and then said, "I'm beginning to see what you're talking about." He would never put Victoria through such an experience.

I found more examples of the pressure Kevin experienced as we talked more about his adult years. Even when his life was going wonderfully, his parents continued to hold back their approval. They expressed disappointment when he chose not to go to law school. They also disagreed with his career in advertising. However, with Jo's love and support, Kevin did not accept their judgments as he had in the past. Then he admitted he resented his parents, which was another clue that Kevin's pain attacks — which began soon after his marriage to Jo — were likely a physical expression of his anger.

Kevin was still not completely convinced. I looked for more evidence that Kevin's childhood had been difficult enough to produce his symptoms. I pointed out that few children could achieve what he had and that many parents heap praise on their offspring for even minor accomplishments. Kevin commented that Clay raised Victoria that way. Then I asked him how hard he competed to get praise from Jo and he began nodding his head that he understood. Jo appreciated him just for waking up in the morning. Kevin then held his face in his hands.

After a few minutes, he looked up and said, "I'm just remembering my wedding reception. My parents were almost rude to Jo. Jo is a hundred times better than the next best thing that ever happened to me and they couldn't even be sociable with her. The thought crossed my mind to throw them out of the reception hall."

The main message to Kevin during his early years, repeated endlessly, was that he did not measure up to expectations. During many of the years needed to unlearn this lesson, he used drugs to ease the emotional pain. Fortunately, he was able to build a more accurate impression of his self-worth by listening to friends, to colleagues at work and later to Jo. As he recognized the magnitude of the harm he suffered as a child, anger and resentment began to build, but he was unaware of the strength of these feelings and unable to put them into words. Physical symptoms were the result.

I recommended he write a letter (not to be mailed) to his parents that included all his thoughts and feelings about their relationship in light of what we had discussed. I offered to refer him for counseling. He made excellent progress in understanding the issues we discussed. His pain attacks quickly ended. Most importantly, he came to see his parents' criticism as a sign of their inadequacy and not his own.

TREATMENT OF CHILDHOOD STRESS

There is only one way to prove that stress is causing an illness: relieve the symptoms by treating the stress. I have tried a variety of treatment techniques and settled on a few that have the greatest practical value. When I see significant improvement in a patient's symptoms, I can be much more confident the diagnosis of stress illness is correct. This enables me to avoid endless diagnostic tests and, when necessary, supports a recommendation that my patient see a mental health counselor.

To overcome childhood stress it is essential to recognize that each of us is vulnerable to accepting false ideas as true, particularly when we are children. In dysfunctional homes, children often learn that they are:

- Unworthy of love, approval or attention
- Unable to measure up to expected standards
- Incapable of having the boundaries of their body respected
- Powerless to change their environment
- Obligated to solve every problem

For the child and later the adult, these false concepts can become fundamental assumptions. To recover from childhood stress it is essential to replace false beliefs with a true understanding of personal strengths and weaknesses. This is rarely easy and can be a daunting task at first. However, many patients feel encouraged when they realize that making this change will not be as difficult as surviving their early years. How does a person develop a more accurate understanding of their self-worth? Start with the following ideas:

1. *Appreciate Your Heroism.* Recognize that merely surviving a dysfunc-

tional childhood is worthy of respect. People often minimize the difficulties they have overcome. When they can appreciate that reaching adulthood required heroic levels of courage and persistence, then they have a foundation for self-esteem. When survivors can take pride in what they have overcome, they begin to unshackle themselves from the past.

> ## Exercise: List of Childhood Stresses
>
> Make a list of every stress you can recall from your childhood. Consider asking siblings and childhood friends to help you remember. Then write about how these events made you feel then and now.

Another idea is to think about other people who have survived difficult experiences. For example, consider someone who has fought in the military or rescued people trapped in a burning building. These people are heroes. But so are survivors of childhood stress because they, too, have overcome serious physical or emotional challenges. The problem is that dysfunctional childhood survivors find it difficult to think of themselves as heroes. Their self-esteem is often too low to accept this idea. Nevertheless, over time, appreciation for what a survivor has accomplished can grow steadily and false self-concepts will fade.

Shauna, age twenty-six, is a good example. As part of my evaluation of her abdominal pains, we discussed her childhood. Shauna told me that at age nine she came to the grim realization that, "If I let my father molest me he would not beat my little brothers as often." After that, she no longer tried to resist his sexual abuse.

After Shauna's statement, I was too shocked to respond right away. I could not imagine how a nine-year-old could have the courage to make such a decision. Usually I try to remain calm and objective when I listen to my patients because it makes difficult questions easier to answer. Shauna's remark left me staring helplessly at the wall. She broke the silence by saying, "I felt so ashamed."

Shauna felt shame about her behavior, instead of awe at her sacrifice. It was clear that she would need to see a counselor regularly, but I wanted to give her something that would support the changes I hoped she would make. On the back of my business card, I wrote, "Shauna is a Hero!" I explained that, like a soldier who saves a comrade under fire or a Coast Guard rescue jumper who plunges into a stormy sea to save a sailor, she had put herself in harm's way to help others. She had also done this for years as a child without any of the advantages of the professional: she had no training, no moral support from comrades, no respite from the physical harm, no ability to fight back, no counseling and no choice.

Shauna taped the card to her bathroom mirror so she could see it every day. I recommended she leave it there until she no longer needed a reminder of her courage. I have since given these Hero Awards to many people to help them reconsider their response to the past. With counseling, Shauna was able to see that her circumstances and her courage dictated her choice and there was no moral failure on her part.

After five years of therapy, Shauna's physical symptoms were improved but still present. She returned to my office hoping that additional diagnostic testing might uncover a visible disease. When these studies were normal, she returned to her counselor with renewed determination to overcome her problems. Her progress has taken time, but Shauna's pain is fading along with her shame.

Shauna's story is a reminder that many people need years of hard work to overcome the injuries of the past. One of my patients remained ill after twelve years of treatment by an excellent mental health counselor. I asked her if she ever felt like giving up. She replied, "Most of the time, no, and I don't get down on myself. Remember, I used to go to the doctor almost every week and I'd be in the hospital several times a year. Now I see the doctor five or ten times a year and I never need the hospital. You showed me how to get better and that gave me hope. I'm okay as long as I keep making progress."

Exercise: The Hero Award

Make a Hero Award for yourself. As you write the words, think about why they are true. Some of my patients find it helpful to make a list of every difficulty they have endured or every experience they might like to change before they make their award. Put the card where you will see it every day. Keep the card until you no longer need it as a reminder.

2. *Understand Connections Between Past and Present.* Our childhood environment teaches us about our world and ourselves. In a healthy environment, we form an accurate self-image and learn constructive habits. In a dysfunctional home, we learn behaviors and beliefs that help us survive, but later these can do more harm than good as in the following examples:

- A person who coped with their early years by working hard to please others might, as an adult, lack experience in caring for themselves. Consequently, they tend to neglect their own needs in favor of taking care of others.
- Children raised without respect are likely to find themselves in disrespectful relationships as adults.
- Children growing up without praise find it difficult to be satisfied with their accomplishments even when others praise their work.
- Some adults cope with trauma from their early years with alcohol or drug abuse, eating disorders or self-mutilation to ease the pain.
- The emotional pain from a difficult childhood can cause depression, anxiety, suicide attempts or other mental health disorders.

Many adults who struggle with these issues view them as personal shortcomings and feel ashamed. I look at them as common consequences of a damaging environment, and try to persuade my patients there is no reason to feel shame about them. I often ask adults who grew up in dysfunctional homes to imagine they were born in a wilderness and had to find their way out before becoming an adult. This analogy emphasizes that they had no responsibility for the harsh environment they found themselves in and that they deserve tremendous credit for having survived.

When patients can leave shame behind, they are one step closer to understanding that the abuse they suffered does not reflect badly on who they are. They can see themselves as good people who began life in a bad place. This is a foundation for self-esteem, which is essential for overcoming illness caused by childhood stress. It is also the first step toward becoming the person they were always meant to be.

3. *Express Emotions Verbally.* As self-esteem grows, so will resentment, anger or anxiety about the childhood mistreatment. If these emotions express themselves as nerve signals traveling into the body, stress illness can result. The next step in treatment is to translate these emotions into words, either written or spoken. Expressing emotions in words reduces expression through the body.

An obstacle to this for some people is that the strength or even the existence of these feelings is not obvious. This is because children bottle up their emotions to help cope with stress and that deprives them of experience feeling and expressing emotions. A person must become aware of an emotion before they can talk about it. Finding a way to more fully perceive these feelings is therefore of key importance. For some patients this is not difficult. All they need is a discussion about their symptoms, a review of their childhood stress and an explanation of the possible connection. This discussion can sometimes produce a revelation that alleviates the symptoms almost immediately. This is what happened to Ellen. Once she found the source of her emotional tension, even driving through Mapleton on the way to visiting her mother lost its power to make her ill.

More commonly, even after talking about childhood stress patients may remain uncertain about the strength of their emotions and the connection to their illness. These people benefit from one or more additional approaches.

One of these techniques is speaking to a mental health counselor. A therapist's training and experience can offer invaluable guidance in understanding the link between past events and present problems.

Another approach involves writing (some individuals get equal benefit from speaking into a recording device). Cecilia is an example of the value of this technique. She was a successful sales professional and motivational speaker, afflicted for many years with a spastic colon. She accessed a number of Internet sites about her condition and usually came to my office armed with new suggestions for diagnosis and treatment.

At each visit for nearly two years, we negotiated as she attempted to "sell" me on which test she should have or which medication should be prescribed. Sometimes I agreed with her. However, her father abused her as a child so I always recommended she write a letter to him that expressed her deepest thoughts and feelings. I failed to make a sale with this suggestion during many, many encounters. Eventually, Cecilia came up with a compromise.

"Dr. Clarke, I'm willing to make a deal with you. I will write two paragraphs to my father if you promise you'll stop asking me to write to him," she said.

"With everything you told me about your father I'm not sure two paragraphs will be enough to help you," I replied.

"Take it or leave it," she said with a smile.

I could see this was the best I could do for her and agreed to the deal. Cecilia lived up to her part of the bargain and wrote the two paragraphs. Then she wrote a third and a fourth. Then, like Dan, the dam burst. By the time the letter was done, it was ten single-spaced typewritten pages. She keeps the letter in a locked desk drawer to this day. Cecilia's symptoms improved by 90 percent and now she manages them with simple treatments and without further tests.

Writing a letter (rarely mailed) to the parent(s) or other individuals who caused stress during childhood is a powerful therapeutic technique though some patients, like Cecilia, need weeks or months to think about it before they are ready. Writing has an almost magical ability to pull buried thoughts and emotions into conscious awareness, which can be very beneficial for stress illness symptoms.

I never ask patients to show me their letters. However, a few patients have shared them and Hope's letter below is a remarkable example. When I met

Hope, she smiled often, laughed easily and did not seem stressed at all. Had we met in a social situation, it would have been easy to assume her life had been a good one from infancy onwards. I have the same impression of many of my stress illness patients.

Hope's illness occurred only at times of stress with her family or at work, but this was several times each month. She had abdominal cramps, diarrhea, nausea, occasional vomiting, felt hot or cold and suffered from anxiety attacks, fatigue and depression. She was twenty-seven and had suffered from these problems since her early teens. However, Hope's physical symptoms were only the beginning of her problems. Every day, physicians evaluate patients like her and never suspect the powerful feelings beneath the surface. Even after several conversations familiarized me with her past, I was stunned at the depth of emotion in her letter. Writing did not immediately relieve Hope's symptoms although she felt much better afterwards. Eventually she recovered completely from her illness. In her letter, only the names and a few identifying details have been changed.

Dear Dad,

All I ever did was love you. I'm tired of being sick. All I ever did was look up to you. I'm tired of being sick. Even through your violent, abusive outbursts, your physical and severe emotional outbursts, your drunkenness, your cussing and name-calling, your bullying and your constant put downs I loved you and I'M TIRED OF BEING SICK!!! I tried to make up for the things, or should I say faults, you found in my mother so you could be happy. I cleaned and I cooked for you. I mowed the grass, did yard work, washed the cars, folded the laundry, made the beds – all because I wanted you to be happy. If you were happy then we could be "abuse-free" for a day. I worked hard – harder than any other child I knew – all to please you. But I never could please you for very long. I'm tired of being sick. I soon realized that I never had a chance at getting my "good" dad back until you stopped drinking so I even tried to remedy that. Of course I couldn't stop you from drinking, but I was willing to try. BECAUSE I AM TIRED OF BEING SICK!

I've been sick for as long as I can remember and I'm just plain tired. I've fought forever and now I'm tired of that too. It's funny to think that even now I look up to you – and I don't have the foggiest idea why. You've put me down in just about every way imaginable. I think you've probably called me every name in the book all strung together for emphasis. You've beat my mother, thrown and broke things in our house, you've jeopardized our safety and our lives, you've left us witness to horrible, outlandish, childish temper tantrums that sorely embarrassed us and our family – and yet despite all of that – we have still loved you and wanted to provide you with happiness. Do you know how many times I've told myself how incredibly stupid I must be for still loving you. You have beaten me down worse than you would to a dog – yet stupid me still looked up to you. Now as an adult I live in constant fear that I may turn out to be as bad a parent as you were. Even though I do nothing the way you do it I am constantly terrified that I just might start. I see the terror reflected in other things also – I can't drink hardly at all. I'm too afraid I'll turn into the monster I swore I would never be – you Dad! I've realized that much of the time I live in constant fear that I can barely keep under the surface. I experience or at least am reminded of that terror every day of my life. I hate to lose control because if I do then I'm no better than my dad. Living in fear is such a shitty way to live. I'm constantly terrified that I am going to screw my marriage up too, just like you and mom did. I know in the end you two managed to work it out and that's an amazing accomplishment yet through the process we children were never protected. I'm so sensitive to Matthew's and my relationship that I can't stand the idea of him being mad at me. If he is mad I live in fear that he will divorce me. I'm tired of being sick. I have so many questions I would love for you to answer yet I know you probably never will. Why did you hurt me so much? I was your child. I needed your love and protection, your guidance and compassion, your instruction and nurturing.

I know at some point you gave me all of these things – the problem is that they got forgotten in the terrible violence and abuse

I encountered on a daily basis. You are such a coward – mom was right and there have been so many times that I have hated you and wished I never had to see you again. You have hurt me worse than any one else ever could. You have damaged me. Being sick is a constant reminder that I am "damaged goods" and yet I have managed to pick myself up time and time again. I have survived you Dad. I have lived in the midst of a 27-year-old storm and been able to come out on the other side. I AM A HERO! I see it every day in my children's eyes. They look at me just the same exact way I looked up to you on several occasions – the difference being they will never have to view me as a violent abuser – they will never slink away or have to live in their rooms in fear of me. I will never break their hearts or tell them what a "dirty rotten piece of shit" they are. I AM A HERO. I have survived you dad. I'm tired of being sick. I'm tired of being in fear. I'm tired of constantly feeling like I have to do more and be the best or everybody might see me as I really perceive myself as "damaged goods" or the "poor abused girl." I hide it all behind a thick layer of self-confidence – yet I'm not really sure if anyone is buying into the cover-up. I know that I still have work to do, but I have made it to the other side. You won't beat me dad   I have won. You have caused me a lot of pain and hours of suffering, but you sonofabitch have not beaten me down. You have not won. Nor will I ever let you. Stop haunting me. 27 years is enough! ENOUGH! I'M TIRED OF BEING SICK!!!

Hope

Writing thoughts and emotions in a journal is another useful technique. A regular log of your ideas will form a record of your progress. In the future if you re-read some of your earlier writing, it can show how far you have come in understanding key issues.

Sometimes it can be helpful to write about certain imaginary situations. For example, think about overhearing a conversation between a parent you do not know and their young child. Through the eavesdropping, you learn that the child is having an experience reminiscent of your own. Then record your ideas and emotional reactions to hearing this. You might find you get quite emotional or feel a strong inclination to lecture the parent.

This actually happened to Paul. He was thirty-one and an optometrist and had grown up in the rural Midwest. His parents had verbally abused him almost from birth. Then at age sixteen, Paul realized he was gay and informed his parents. They brought him to church and placed him in a chair at the front. His friends and relatives came to the pulpit one after another and demanded that Paul change his ways. They told him he was "evil" and "sinful." Eighteen months later, his father died suddenly and the family blamed Paul for his death. Estrangement from his family was now complete and he left for the nearest big city to attend college.

Paul held deep anger within him that no one ever observed, which showed itself only as severe headaches. When he began a close and supportive relationship with a new partner, these became much worse, (an example of the Good Partner/Bad Illness syndrome). One day in a bookstore, he overheard a woman verbally abusing her eight-year-old son. It was a strong reminder of how his parents had treated him.

Something snapped in Paul and he walked over to the woman in a blind rage. He erupted in front her and let her know very clearly, in a way she would not soon forget, that her behavior was damaging to her son. Paul had no explanation for his reaction until we discussed the connection to his childhood. I recommended that he explore his anger through writing and with a counselor. His headaches improved steadily.

4. *Mental Health Counseling.* Most patients, but not all, will respond well to use of the methods described above. Particularly for my readers who are not making progress with other treatment techniques described in this section or those who have significant mental health problems, psychiatric intervention can be a key to recovery from stress illness. *Be aware that counselors vary in their experience and interest in childhood stress issues.* If these are the problems of greatest concern, be sure the counselor treats people for this regularly. You should also be aware that drug or alcohol abuse reduces success rates and needs treatment at the same time as the stress illness.

5. *Self-Care.* A technique described in more detail in the chapter on current stress can also help survivors of childhood stress. Spend five to six hours each week entirely in self-care. Many childhood stress survivors never learned how to play. Taking time for personal recreation is an act of self-care that can be an important foundation for self-esteem. Through recreation, people teach themselves they are worthy of caring.

6. *Other Useful Techniques.* Many of my patients experience difficulty connecting with emotions appropriate for their childhood experience. Here is an exercise that can help.

Exercise: Identify a Child

Begin by thinking of a child whom you know and care about. (If you do not know any children, go to an elementary school at recess and focus for a moment on a child who reminds you of yourself.) Then imagine this child is experiencing the same stresses you did when you were young. Imagine you are able to witness these problems, but not able to intervene. Write about how this makes you feel. Write what you would like to say to the child to help them survive the experience. For many survivors of child abuse, this is the most important exercise in this book.

If a person feels comfortable discussing these issues in front of others then a support group can be helpful. Support groups might be available through churches, some YWCAs and Alcoholics Anonymous. The latter often includes groups for Adult Children of Alcoholics and these can be helpful for anyone from a dysfunctional family even if your parents were not alcoholic. If you cannot find a group, the United Way, a social worker or librarian might be able to help you.

Some communities or large health maintenance organizations have classes for Adult Children of Alcoholics and Dysfunctional Families. Typically, these are small groups, and those who take part are themselves an important source of information for their classmates.

Another resource is books about recovery from childhood stress. When I began working in this field in the 1980s, there were very few helpful books available but now they are abundant. See Appendix I for several excellent references.

Recovery from childhood stress is frequently difficult and painful, can take a long time and requires persistence. There are no easy answers, but confidence gained from having already survived difficult problems will ensure eventual success.

CHAPTER 4
CURRENT STRESS

Anyone who wishes to combine domestic responsibilities and paid employment with the least stress and most enjoyment might start by pondering this paradox: the first step to better functioning is to stop blaming herself for not functioning well enough.

– Faye J. Crosby

CURRENT STRESS: KENDALL

With one exception, Kendall was convinced she had everything under control. She was thirty-three and a paralegal at a large law firm downtown. This was her dream job. She worked hard to put herself through school and get the grades and academic honors that earned her the position three years before. Now her job performance was in jeopardy because of one item she could not manage: months of severe back and chest pain occasionally accompanied by nausea. Tests done by her primary care doctor returned entirely normal.

After she learned about the ability of stress to cause illness, I asked if there were any unusual difficulties recently.

"Not really," she replied. "I love my job. My marriage is good and I have a great family."

I remained suspicious that she was coping with more stress than she realized because her tests had shown no other explanation for her symptoms.

"Can you give me some more details about your daily routine?" I asked.

She worked forty to forty-five hours each week. Her husband, a nurse supervisor, worked during the evening shift. They saw each other only briefly during the week. When Kendall arrived home in the evening, her six children who ranged from toddler to teen were there to greet her. Another of Kendall's responsibilities was caring for her father who had a serious degenerating nerve disease. He not only lived in Kendall's home but, at times, he needed almost as much care as one of the children.

Kendall was managing her full-time job, six children, her household and a disabled father. She had done this for so many years that it seemed quite normal to her. However, when you are on a treadmill like that with no opportunity to stop and take a break, chances are your body will protest eventually. When she finished describing her life, I just looked at her and said, "Wow." She understood my diagnosis immediately and started to laugh. "I forgot to tell you I also do a lot of volunteer work at the community center," she said and smiled as my shoulders slumped. Just listening to her describe everything she accomplished each week was almost enough to cause *my* chest to start hurting.

I recommended five hours every week of self-care time, but she was reluctant. She had been hoping for treatment with medication or a procedure. Kendall also had no idea how she would find five hours every week, since she assumed her usual responsibilities would simply accumulate until she returned.

It was essential her family take on some household work so she could enjoy this time. Kendall objected that she would probably feel very guilty if she just dropped her work onto others. I pointed out her many responsibilities were likely the cause of her pains. In a way, her body was trying to tell her that her workload was too high.

"If you don't take care of yourself, your body will make it even more difficult for you to do what your family needs," I said.

Since she had not indulged herself for years, Kendall was unsure how she would use the free time. I told her it would take practice and trial and error before she learned what she needed to do.

"When you find yourself looking forward to that time every week, then you will know you are on the right track," I told her. "All I'm asking you to do is put yourself on the list of people you take care of."

Fortunately, her family was sympathetic and gave her their full support. She found she could leave her home on Saturday afternoons and return in the evening without finding unfinished work waiting for her. She used the time in a variety of ways. She went to the library to read. She took long walks or saw a movie with a friend. Another time she went to the zoo. With each activity, she learned a little more about what she needed. It was not long before her Saturday afternoons left her feeling rejuvenated. Within a few months, her symptoms disappeared.

CURRENT STRESS: SHARON

Sharon was an athletic thirty-one-year-old mother of two who suffered an attack of severe abdominal pain a few hours before we met. When it did not let up, she came to the emergency room where she needed narcotic injections for relief. She told the emergency room physician the pain "feels like my lymph nodes again." She experienced similar pain thirteen years earlier in her small hometown in eastern Washington, spending three weeks in the hospital and undergoing a large number of tests. Finally, her doctors concluded the lymph nodes in her abdomen were inflamed. Toward the end of the three weeks, her pain went away, not returning until now.

This time though, the location of her pain, the findings on her examination and several diagnostic studies showed no evidence of lymph node inflammation or any other serious abdominal condition. This led me to think about the possibility of stress illness.

Sharon turned out to be a busy woman. In addition to caring for her children (aged nine and eleven), she worked full time, as did her husband. Both children were competitive springboard divers and Sharon took them to practice early in the morning and often in the evening as well. Most weekends there were more practices or competitions and the latter might be many hours away by car. Sharon was also part of the swim club board of directors and was a diving coach for her children and others.

"Do you get much personal time?" I asked.

"Personal time? What's that?" she laughed. "Maybe once in a while I'll go to a movie with my husband. I guess I just like being busy. Even when I was a kid I used to dive before school, after school and on weekends."

Her diving career began at age four. She never really had time to play like other girls her age. In high school, her father apologized to her because he felt he had pushed her too hard.

"I won a national AAU championship in high school," she continued. "But after that I decided enough was enough." She stopped practicing and never entered another competition. She admitted she felt completely burned out. A few weeks after this great victory she was in the hospital with abdominal pain.

I wondered about the timing of her earlier illness. Perhaps it had not been due to her lymph nodes, but to the stress of giving up diving after so many years of intense involvement. She remembered there had been great difficulty diagnosing the cause of her pain. Near the end of three weeks in the hospital, as her illness was finishing its course, the doctors told her their diagnosis but without conclusive proof.

As we talked she began feeling better even though she had not had a narcotic injection for many hours. This was reassuring evidence she did not have a serious abdominal disease. If she had stress illness instead, what would alleviate her stress?

Sharon, so dedicated to diving as a child, never had enough opportunities to play. She knew a great deal about self-sacrifice, but not enough about her own limits, about taking care of herself and about everyone's need for relaxation and self-care. She took care of everyone else so much she forgot herself. Her pain was due to her body protesting. She needed to learn how to give herself a break.

As with Kendall, I recommended Sharon set aside five hours each week when someone else would manage all her usual responsibilities. Her husband was confident the family could arrange this. When I asked Sharon if she felt she could do this she asked a revealing question: "But what would I do during that time?" I hear this question often from my patients who need to learn how to care for themselves. They find it difficult to think of pleasurable ways to use their free time.

I advised Sharon to use trial and error to find activities so enjoyable she would look forward to them every week. "Learning how to use this time will be like learning a new dive. You won't get it exactly right at first, but you will improve," I assured her. She went home from the emergency room with additional pain medication, my office phone number in case the symptoms worsened and a follow-up appointment. Two weeks later, her pain was much less severe, but still present.

I asked about her progress with personal time. She had first taken time to relax the day after I saw her in the emergency room. She curled up in a recliner with a good book while her family cleaned house. For the next fifteen minutes, she felt intensely guilty. When she could not endure it any longer, she went to the kitchen and began cleaning up even though her family urged her to return to her chair. The second week she did a little better, but still found it difficult to take a break.

"Your body is using the pain to let you know you need more practice taking care of yourself," I explained. I reassured her she was off to a good start and that guilt was normal at the beginning. Afterward, she made good progress learning how to relax and enjoy herself. She began taking long walks in a nearby park. During one of those walks, she remembered she always found listening to a piano to be relaxing. She found a teacher and began taking lessons. Within six weeks, she had no more pain.

CURRENT STRESS: NANCY

Taking time for self-care seems like it should be such an easy thing to do. But often there are hidden forces that undermine our best intentions. Nancy had abdominal symptoms for years, dozens of negative diagnostic tests and an endlessly busy lifestyle that gave her no time for self-care. Unfortunately, Nancy had even more difficulty using time for enjoyment than Sharon did. Even with the support of her family and weeks of trying, she could not find a way to relax and have fun. Nearly two months after we discussed personal self-care, she drove off from home planning to do something enjoyable, but couldn't think of anything and ended up buying groceries and having the tires rotated.

For Nancy, the concept of self-care represented a major change in lifestyle. In the small number of my patients who are unable to make this change, I try to find the reasons. If I can do that, I usually can find a way to help people make progress.

Nancy grew up as one of the middle children in a large family. Dad was an alcoholic, Mom was angry a lot and Nancy spent her childhood unsuccessfully trying to make things better. She remembered searching the house for her father's hidden liquor bottles. After finding one, she poured the contents down a drain then returned the bottle to its hiding place with a short note so her father would know who was responsible. He never said a word to her about this.

While growing up, Nancy did not mention or even think about her own needs very often. Taking care of everyone else and doing whatever her siblings wanted to do was her normal way of life. She had far fewer opportunities for carefree play than most children did. Consequently, Nancy never learned how to care for herself. As an adult, she attended to everyone else in her world but rarely took time for her own needs. This is a common outcome for many people who grew up in difficult circumstances. Nancy did not perceive a significant problem with this as a child or as an adult. For years, her husband had urged her to do more for herself, but she could always think of something more "useful" to do.

Nancy had an eight-year-old daughter named April. I asked Nancy if April spent time playing without thinking about the needs of others. "Of course she does," Nancy replied.

"Nancy, would it bother you if April spent most of her time taking care of other family members like you did when you were her age?" I asked.

Nancy replied immediately, "I wouldn't want that for my daughter."

"Then imagine for a moment that April was growing up in a family exactly like the one you grew up in. Suppose you had to watch April in that environment but you couldn't do anything to help her."

Nancy quickly became emotional. The thought of April enduring the same troubles Nancy had struggled with as a child made it clear how difficult her environment had been. This painful image helped Nancy to see how her problems caring for herself grew out of the neglect she suffered when she was young. If neglecting April would be a problem now, so was neglecting Nancy back then. If letting April play was a good thing, it might be good for Nancy, too.

With these ideas in mind Nancy was able to use April's carefree playing as a model. When she returned for her next office visit, she was a different person. Her husband received a significant raise in salary and she seized this opportunity to take a six-month leave of absence from her job so she could "find myself." Once she made this decision, over ten years of physical symptoms vanished.

CURRENT STRESS: MORGAN

Morgan's illness began in his church. He was a forty-six-year-old native of Tennessee who worked in the horticulture industry in Oregon. He possessed a slight southern accent and a sophisticated vocabulary, and was the only member of his family with a college education. I had helped him with his heartburn a few years before, but now he was back with a new problem.

There was a small area of his abdomen (just below the ribs on the left side) that developed moderate amounts of pain a few times each month. The pain would last for several hours and then vanish. Another symptom was tightness in his throat. This was sometimes strong enough to interfere with swallowing. That sensation, too, would go away in a few hours. Both of these symptoms began about a year before.

Based on his description, it seemed likely that these symptoms resulted from tightening of the muscles of his gastrointestinal tract. Spasm of the large intestine would account for the abdominal pain and spasm of the esophagus for the throat problem. Stress is often responsible for gastrointestinal muscle tightening. I asked him if there had been any difficulties in his life over the last year.

Morgan displayed little emotion. With no change in the tone of his voice, he began to talk about his church. He had been on the board of directors and taught four or five different Bible study classes. Morgan was also heavily involved in fundraising so the church could expand the building in which they met for services.

This situation began to go wrong for him just before his symptoms started. Two members of the board of directors opposed expanding the building. As senior members of two large, extended families that together made up nearly half of the church membership, they succeeded in uniting these families behind an effort that blocked the fundraising. Morgan commented, "Politics like that has no place in the church." As he prayed about what to do, he cried.

This was not the end of Morgan's difficulties. He resigned from the board because they ignored his views or voted them down. The board stripped him of all but one of his Bible classes. They appointed a deacon from one of the two large families who opposed the fundraising. This deacon would be nearly impossible to remove from this position and became a strong influence on the pastor. When this happened, Morgan again prayed about what to do. He became so angry he could not cry. He was now deliberating whether to leave the church, but the pastor asked him to stay. In spite of his strong feelings, Morgan said all of this in the same tone he might have used to describe a trip to buy groceries. Perhaps the emotions were going to his esophagus and large intestine instead.

I explained how high levels of stress could cause the mind to send nerve signals into the body. "When these signals arrive, muscle spasm results," I told him. It was likely that his symptoms would continue until he found a resolution to his difficulties with the church. He was reassured that his symptoms were not likely to be signs of a serious problem. I recommended he continue to pray and that he return if the problems changed or worsened. I was confident he would find a solution to the dilemma and that when he did the symptoms would improve.

I telephoned him two months later. He left the church with great regret, but found a new one that welcomed him. He was teaching Bible study again and attendance was growing as the congregation became aware of his gifts as a teacher. His pains were gone.

CURRENT STRESS: CARLA

Carla came to my office with a two-quart pot into which she spit up small amounts of fluid throughout the appointment. She seemed badly in need of a rest. Relieving her symptoms would prove to be one of the most difficult challenges of my career but, except for the pot, there was no way to anticipate that from her appearance.

She was twenty-four, quite tall (which suited her high school career as a basketball player) and six months pregnant. Carla vomited many days every year for the last seven years, though very little in the first three months of her pregnancy, which is when morning sickness is most common. Suddenly, in the last three weeks, her vomiting began occurring every day even though she limited her diet. Her blood pressure and pulse revealed evidence of dehydration.

It was possible that her symptoms were due to an obstruction of her stomach or intestine. I admitted her to the hospital for intravenous fluids and a video exam of her stomach. This was normal except for the presence of vegetable fiber, still in her stomach twenty-four hours after ingestion. An x-ray showed no evidence of obstruction of her bowels.

After I ran several more tests, the most likely remaining explanation for her symptoms was sluggish or weak contraction of the muscles of her stomach. This would result in food not getting to the intestine, causing the stomach to overfill, which results in vomiting. A sluggish stomach occurs most often in older patients who have nerve disease or long-standing diabetes, but is rare in an otherwise healthy young woman.

I gave Carla high doses of medications intended to get her stomach moving and relieve nausea. Her vomiting did not improve. She remained in the hospital, unable to keep down broth, sports drinks or even water. Could stress cause such a dramatic change in physiology?

Carla and Matt had been happily married for several years. She enjoyed her work as a salesperson in a furniture store. She had some symptoms of depression including fatigue. Recently she noticed that minor issues in her work and at home were causing much more distress than usual. Whether these symptoms were truly due to depression or simply to the emotional drain of her repeated vomiting was not clear. Another of Carla's qualities, strong Christian faith that she rarely mentioned in casual conversation, proved to be important later on.

When she was three, her parents divorced and she lived with her father. Her mother never remarried and lived only a few towns away, but never had any contact with Carla, not even so much as a holiday card or birthday present.

Carla and Matt fell in love when they were teenagers. While both were still in high school, she became pregnant. An agonizing review of their options led to a decision to give the baby up for adoption. A few years later, they married. Now several years after their wedding, she was pregnant for the second time.

Carla did not speak easily about her feelings. However, seeing her daily in the hospital helped me get to know her better. I began to sense she had strong emotions barely under control. She seemed particularly emotional about her mother, Virginia. Why had this woman abandoned Carla? What reason could there be for cutting off all contact with your only daughter? As one diagnostic test after another proved to be normal, I decided to explore the idea of re-uniting mother and daughter. Carla was willing to let me telephone Virginia, though she had never done so herself. She also agreed to meet her mother.

There were many ways in which this could go wrong, but I was running out of ideas. Fortunately, on the phone Virginia seemed to be a decent woman who was quite concerned to learn that Carla was in the hospital. She agreed to pay a visit. The next day I came to see Carla in the afternoon and learned that her mother spent the whole morning with her. Their conversation could not have gone better. They cleared up two decades of misunderstandings and agreed to see each other again regularly. Even better, Carla was ready to try some lunch.

Lunch stayed down. So did dinner, then breakfast. This was the first time in a month that Carla could digest food. I sent Carla home, to her great relief and mine. Resolving her dilemma kept me elated for about six weeks, right up to the moment I learned that Carla was back in the hospital with vomiting and dehydration.

My first thought was something had happened between Carla and her mother. But the time they spent together after Carla left the hospital had gone well. I reviewed all her tests to see if we had missed anything. I looked again into my textbooks for obscure diseases that can cause vomiting. I searched the Internet and the medical literature databases. I reviewed the case with a colleague at a university. None of this produced anything useful.

I prescribed an antidepressant medicine without much hope it would help. I questioned her again about how things were going with Virginia. Were there still issues of resentment? Carla was reasonably sure there were none and was optimistic about the prospects for building a good relationship.

All my assumptions about the nature of her illness were now in disarray. I thought about referring her to the university for another opinion. I thought about sending her home with nutrition provided by a tube placed in a large vein inside her chest. I began to think about her most of the time.

This is a good example of how my patients have taught me about stress illness. When their symptoms do not improve, I have either not under-

stood their stresses well enough or I have not designed a treatment program that meets their needs. At this stage of my work with Carla, I had
problems in both areas. Unfortunately, there is no cookbook for stress illness diagnosis and no recipe for treatments that will always work. During
encounters with thousands of patients, a combination of careful listening
and trial and error has enabled me to find the most practical techniques for
relieving symptoms.

As I thought about Carla, one fact began to stand out: for six weeks after
leaving the hospital, she was well and her improvement immediately followed
the meeting with her mother. If this was not a coincidence, then her symptoms must have improved because of psychological factors. Therefore, her
relapse might be due to a psychological factor, but one I had not found yet.
Could she possibly have two different stresses capable of paralyzing her stomach? If so, what had I missed?

With these ideas in mind, I reviewed her records from the beginning and
noticed that her vomiting episodes started seven years ago, exactly when she
and Matt had given their infant son up for adoption. I recognized this coincidence earlier, but was distracted from it by the discussion about Virginia.

I went back to the hospital and asked Carla to talk about her son. She told
me her pregnancy before marriage conflicted with her strong religious principles. The decision to have her son adopted was the most painful of her life.
She had no contact with her son and no knowledge of his whereabouts, yet
thought about him frequently.

"Whenever I'm in a crowd, I look at the faces of boys who are about his
age and wonder if one of them is him," she said sadly. She felt guilty for having abandoned her son just as her mother had abandoned her. But was this
enough to paralyze a stomach?

No, there was more. It was not easy for Carla to discuss, but her guilt was
deeper than what she felt for repeating Virginia's desertion. For Carla, having
a child outside of marriage and then giving him up for adoption were terrible
sins against God. She believed in the concept of divine retribution and for
the last seven years had lived with a small but constant fear she would suffer
punishment. She and Matt tried to conceive another child for several years
without success until now. Since her first pregnancy occurred easily, Carla in-

terpreted the long wait for the second pregnancy as part of her punishment.

After a long conversation, it became clear she had an even greater concern. Perhaps a fitting retribution for her "sin" would be for her second child to have serious birth defects. Carla's fears about what might lie ahead for her unborn child grew directly in parallel with her enlarging womb. She was now just six weeks from her due date. Carla's fear was barely under control. Her inability to comprehend or fully express this verbally left her needing to express it physically through vomiting.

Our discussion enabled her to put her anxiety into words for the first time. Unfortunately, her ability to describe these problems was not enough to solve them. Her vomiting persisted. How could her fears be relieved? I thought about how Carla viewed the world and I tried to imagine the emotions she must be experiencing. It seemed likely that Carla's abandonment by Virginia predisposed Carla to assume guilt for negative events in her life. Her guilt about the adoption of her son was so extreme, she believed God would punish her. I looked for a way to help her see these issues more positively.

The next day I asked Carla if she believed God gave Jesus to humanity so that lives would be better. She was clear she did believe this. Then I asked if she had given her son to the adopting parents so they might have better lives. She did not reply, but slowly sat up and shifted her gaze from the floor to the window.

"You suffered when you gave up your son, Carla," I said. "This was a sacrifice you made for his benefit and for his adopting parents. Was that so very different from God giving His Son to mankind?" I paused to let her think about this and then said, "I would like you to think about whether God might look favorably on the choice that you made."

Carla was able to leave the hospital the next day. I am sure the successful reunion with her mother helped Carla accept the idea that the adoption of her son was a sacrifice and not a sin. She gave birth to a healthy child six weeks later. Nine months after the birth I called Matt (Carla was difficult to reach by phone) and he reported the baby was thriving. Matt also told me both he and Carla looked upon their new daughter as a gift from a God who loved their family. There has been no further vomiting.

CURRENT STRESS: JIM

Jim was a middle-aged auto detailer who toughed it out through symptoms that would bring most people to their knees. After his divorce two years earlier Jim had been in the hospital six times for attacks of vomiting. He tried to manage these attacks at home and usually arrived at the emergency room barely able to stand. Diagnostic testing showed no cause for his symptoms. He always improved after a few days. Then he would feel well for a few months until another attack occurred, usually without warning.

Jim's doctor called and told me Jim had waited five days to come to the hospital and his kidneys nearly shut down from lack of fluid. Even worse, he was not responding to treatment the way he had in the past. As usual, tests done to find the cause of his vomiting were normal. When I went to the hospital to see him I found a surprise. Someone had erased his name from the white board that lists patients' names. Instead, next to his room number were the letters "DNA." Oddly enough, this turned out to be the key to his diagnosis.

DNA means "Do Not Announce," which meant telephone callers or visitors would not be told where Jim was staying or even that he was in the hospital. A large, hand-written "No Visitors" sign hung from his door. The only light in the room, dim but colorful, was from a silent television. The scene resembled an empty dance club. Jim was muscular, with thick blond hair and a full beard. He sprawled on the bed with his face half-turned into the pillow. He did not move when I introduced myself.

After he described his symptoms, I asked about the careful protection of his privacy. The story began with Jim's friend Henry. Henry and his wife Gretchen recently divorced and Gretchen had sole custody of their two children. Henry wanted time with his children but Gretchen refused. Jim had been friends with Gretchen in high school so Henry came to Jim asking for help.

Henry, whom Jim described as a "fanatic," came to Jim a lot and refused to leave him alone. Now he had even come to the hospital. Without any regard for his severe illness, he continued to push Jim to intervene with Gretchen on his behalf. Jim was outraged at this invasion of his privacy. Replacing his name on the board with "DNA" and the "No Visitors" sign kept Henry away.

Jim, kind-hearted to a fault, found it impossible to turn down a person in need — no matter how obnoxious. He had to call on the support of hospital privacy policy in order to rid himself of Henry. On his own, he was unable to keep him out of his life.

This episode revealed a great deal about Jim's personality. It was no surprise to learn that he made sacrifices to help a number of individuals and worthy causes. This was in addition to his full-time job, coping with his divorce and parenting two teenaged children.

Jim was capable of handling enormous amounts of stress. But he kept adding so many responsibilities and commitments that now his body was trying to tell him he had taken on too much. We spoke for a long time about how to set limits on how much he would do for others. We discussed managing the guilt he felt when he turned someone down. I advised him to listen to the message his body was sending. I stressed the importance of recognizing that he deserved to be cared for as much as the people who came to him in need.

Jim sat up for the first time. He said, "You might be on to something there." I waited as he sat quietly. Suddenly he grabbed a large basin and began vomiting until he half-filled it. I began to wonder about my diagnosis, but continued to talk to him about strategies for limiting his commitments. Fortunately, by the next morning he felt well, ate a full breakfast and informed his primary physician he was ready to go home.

It was not long before Henry was calling Jim again. But now Jim was able to make it clear he would not help him any further. He told Henry to write to Gretchen and hung up the phone. This success made other changes seem even easier. Soon he found he had time not only to care for his business and his children, but also for himself. He has had no further hospital stays.

The stories in this chapter describe severe levels of stress. Fortunately, the treatments that helped these patients are effective for people coping with a variety of issues. The next section reviews these techniques.

TREATMENT FOR CURRENT STRESSES

I used to believe I would never get stress-related symptoms myself. But every so often, particularly when I am in the hospital and needed for too many bleeding ulcers and obstructed bile ducts, I unconsciously hunch up my shoulders. By late afternoon, they are stiff and sore and I realize I should have followed the advice below on relaxation technique. My patients cope with stress much more often than I do, but they learn to take control and change it for the better. Here are several simple yet effective methods for coping with current stresses.

The Stress Inventory. One of the most useful techniques for managing stress is to list everything that causes you worry, anxiety, fear, tension, anger or emotional pain. Keep the inventory with you so that you can add to it whenever a new idea comes to mind. Many people are quite surprised at the number of items that end up on their list.

Once the inventory seems complete, you can re-write it with the most troubling issues at the top. Next, pick two or three items you can change for the better. If you succeed in making those changes, that might be all you need to see some relief of stress illness symptoms.

The inventory can also clarify connections between particular stresses and your illness. For example, if you notice many items on the list that relate to your job, you might suddenly realize how often your stomach is in knots while commuting to the workplace. The list can also clarify your understanding of which issues have solutions in the short term and which will take longer.

Another benefit is that the act of writing can jump-start your brain into working on solutions. How does this work? Have you ever seen a movie actor that you know you have seen before, but you cannot remember the name of the film? If so, perhaps you have also had the experience, several hours later, of suddenly remembering the forgotten title. This happened because your brain was stimulated to work on the problem "in the background" while you went about your day. The stress inventory can work the same way. You might not see many solutions at first, but your brain will be stimulated to work on your problems and you will soon find that solutions start to appear.

Jodi was a forty-two-year-old mother of three with tight shoulder muscles and steadily worsening constipation. Her inventory looked something like this:

- Supervisor at work sometimes verbally abusive
- Husband Mark arrives home from work too tired to talk

- She and Mark never seem to get out of the house together without the children
- Jodi's mother-in-law has told the children about items the mother-in-law has shoplifted
- Jodi's father continues to abuse alcohol while her mother simply tolerates it
- Jodi's shoulder tension is worse in the later afternoon and early evening as she tries to finish work, get home and prepare dinner

After our discussion, Jodi understood these issues could be an important cause of her illness. She also accepted responsibility for making changes. She succeeded in setting aside time after supper to share her day with her husband. She arranged one evening out with him every week or two. She persuaded her husband to speak to his mother about her behavior. She began teaching her children to help prepare meals. She was not ready to confront her supervisor or her father, but was "working on that, too." Her shoulders and her bowels improved considerably because of these changes.

Setting Limits. Many of my patients take care of everyone that needs them before they consider their own needs. No human being can sustain this indefinitely and eventually the body will protest. To prevent this, consider the ideas in the box about setting limits.

Exercise: How to Set Limits

- If you have not done so already, make a list of all the difficulties you have overcome in your life starting in childhood. Reviewing this list should help you feel justified spending more time on what truly matters to you. You might find it difficult to set limits until you believe you have earned the right to care for yourself.

- Make a list of all your current commitments. This might include family, friends, job, community organizations and hobbies.

- Circle items on the commitments list that have the lowest importance to you.

- Write a specific plan to reduce less important commitments. Jim, for example, wrote down exactly what he would say to Henry to discourage future contact.

Self-Care Time. A third technique for reducing stress is to take five to six hours of personal self-care time every week. This is particularly valuable for my patients who find themselves rarely having any personal time. These people are so busy taking care of family, job and other commitments that they never have time to take care of themselves, as if they live on a stair step machine they cannot stop. Even worse, when they look into the future they see few opportunities for changing this situation.

Taking the whole five to six hours at once usually works best because it gives you enough time to get far away from your other responsibilities. To avoid distraction by unfinished chores, I recommend leaving your home during this time. Others should take responsibility for some of your usual tasks so you can focus on yourself. (You cannot truly enjoy yourself if you are worried about unfinished business at your home or workplace.) You might need support from everyone in the household to get away. To feel better about asking for this support, try to recognize that all you are doing is including yourself among the people you care for.

During this time, you should do something that leaves you fresh and rejuvenated at the end. You can do this alone or with friends or family as long as the time is *all about you.* Many people feel quite guilty at first, but *with practice,* they find it gets easier. To help you let go of the guilt, remind yourself how much time you spend helping others. Your guilt will decline further if stress illness symptoms improve. You can then think of the personal time as a medical prescription. It also helps if you recognize you cannot fulfill your responsibilities if you are ill.

Many individuals who benefit from self-care time never truly learned how to play as children. This could be because they had too many adult responsibilities while young. For others, it was because they grew up in fear, turmoil or neglect. Children in those situations focus on what is going on around them to the exclusion of themselves. As a result, they do not develop a clear sense of their own needs. Taking personal time becomes a foreign concept. *For people in this situation, it is vital to understand that enjoying personal time is an essential human skill.* Fortunately, people who did not learn this as children can acquire the ability at any stage of life.

Many of my patients who need this technique the most have little or no idea what to do with five to six hours of free time. If you are one of these people, let your imagination come up with ideas. Use trial and error. Try to feel or behave like a child. Learning what is pleasurable for you is like learning any new skill. You might not get it completely right at first, but each time you try, you will improve. You will also recognize you not only need this new ability, but you deserve it as well.

Once acquired, you will always have this skill to call upon when needed. You will also have a clearer sense of when your stress level is getting too high. Then you will know how to stop and give yourself a break so the stress does not reach the level of causing illness. Think about the suggestions in the self-care ideas box below to help you get started.

Exercise: Self Care Ideas

- Play with a child
- Exercise: walk, hike, dance, jog, swim, bicycle, learn a new sport (before beginning an exercise program, check with your doctor if you have any reason for concern about your heart or lungs)
- Attend a concert, play, movie or athletic contest
- Share a meal with a friend
- Visit a spa, have a massage or facial, try aromatherapy
- Enjoy a weekend out of town
- Visit a comedy club
- Learn yoga or meditation
- Take lessons in a craft or musical instrument
- If you have a sexual partner, talk with them about adding some variety to your sex life
- Admire or purchase some flowers or artwork
- Read a book or listen to music
- Visit or work in a garden or museum
- Travel to a place you have never seen (it doesn't need to be far away)
- Play a board game with friends
- Work on a puzzle (crossword, sudoku, jigsaw or other type)

I play indoor soccer every Thursday night with a team I have been with since 1990. After a week of mentally demanding work, there is something uniquely satisfying about a good pass or just blasting the ball toward the goal (even though it does not go in as often as I get older). I also enjoy having a beer with the team afterward, particularly since we talk about everything but our work.

Relaxation Technique. A fourth method for reducing stress is relaxation technique. We have seen how the mind can unload stress into the body. However, with just a few minutes of relaxation technique, the body can send a stress-reducing message back to the mind. To understand how this works let me review the body's reaction to stress.

Nerve signals from the stress response system cause rapid, shallow breathing, a fast heartbeat and tense muscles. These reactions evolved to help us run from predators or fight enemies. Today our brain calls upon this same stress response for a variety of situations such as an angry spouse, an unexpectedly large bill or losing your job. The relaxation response balances the stress response. Here the breathing is deeper and slower, the heart rate declines and muscles relax. By initiating this response yourself, you can significantly lower your stress level. Begin by finding a quiet place. Try to ensure no interruptions for ten or twenty minutes. Get into a comfortable position. Pads on the floor, a bed, or a reclining chair are all effective. Dim lights and soft music enhance the experience for many people. Then follow the instructions in the box. For some people the stress level rises steadily during the day as one difficult event after another occurs. Relaxation technique will take only minutes and can bring the stress level down whenever it threatens to get too high. You can use it several times in a day if necessary.

As with any new skill, you could find this difficult at first. Most people improve with practice. Give yourself a few weeks and your sense of control over the stresses in your life should increase significantly. A few people find this technique makes them feel more stressed. If you are one of them, you might be suffering from an anxiety disorder and could benefit from a discussion with a mental health counselor.

Yoga, meditation, prayer or even getting a massage can give similar results. The underlying principle is the same: to deliver a relaxation response message to the brain to bring the stress level down.

Exercise: Relaxation Technique

Place your hands together on the middle of your abdomen. Breathe slowly in and out through your nose, deeply enough so you can feel your hands rise and fall with your abdomen. Once you feel comfortable, close your eyes and imagine a comforting word, phrase or place. (Some people feel more relaxed with their eyes open and so need not close them.)

Next, unless you already feel tension in the muscles around your feet, tense these muscles gently for a few seconds as you inhale slowly, then completely relax the muscles as you exhale. (If you can feel tension in a muscle before you start the exercise you do not need to tense it further.) As you continue to breathe, pay attention to the difference in how the muscles felt during tension and relaxation and try to get them completely relaxed.

Repeat this exercise with the other muscle groups one by one. After your feet do this with the lower legs, the thighs and buttocks, the abdomen, the lower back, the chest, the upper back, the hands and forearms, then the shoulders, the neck and lastly the head. Finally, let your whole body relax for several more breaths to complete the exercise. This technique sends your mind a strong message that all is well and will significantly decrease your stress level.

CHAPTER 5

TRAUMATIC STRESS

*I toyed with the idea of going to find another war where
I could at least feel alive. I was so numb that it took
terror to make me feel anything.*

– Bess Jones, U.S. Army nurse during
the Vietnam War

TRAUMATIC STRESS: AMY

THE KEY TO AMY'S DIAGNOSIS TURNED OUT TO BE A GESTURE SHE MADE WITH HER right hand. For three years, thirty-five-year-old Amy had been afflicted with severe attacks of abdominal pain and vomiting that came on without warning. These would cause her to double over and often required narcotic injections in an emergency room for relief. These episodes occurred three to four times each year and usually persisted for days. The pain always went away as mysteriously and quickly as it had started. Between attacks, she felt perfectly well, but the illness put a terrible strain on her ability to care for her family while she also worked as a receptionist for a dentist.

The many doctors who evaluated her performed a variety of blood tests, x-ray studies and ultrasound imaging. None of these showed any abnormality. After the first two years, her doctors stopped doing diagnostic tests and simply gave her pain relievers.

When I asked her to point out the location of her pain, Amy responded by forming her right hand into the shape used by children who want to pretend they are holding a gun. She pointed the "barrel" at the right lower corner of her abdomen. Most of my patients with abdominal pain tend to place their palm over the painful area. I did not understand the significance of the gesture right away, but later it made perfect sense.

I asked her about stress. She responded that working in the dental office paid the bills, there were no troubling personal relationships and she was devoted to her husband and children. Amy had no significant symptoms of depression or anxiety. Had she experienced any traumatic events in her life?

She replied that when she was a teenager in Minnesota her older brother Tom had died. Amy admired Tom during all her years growing up. However, Amy had never shared the story of his death with any of her friends in Oregon except her husband. What had made her hold back? Her brother had died from a gunshot wound.

Amy was not comfortable telling the story. "It was around Thanksgiving," she began. "Tom and I were at my parents' house and a man Tom knew at work came over. They started drinking beer and then they started arguing. I don't even remember what it was about. They went outside and started fighting. I kept telling them to stop and finally the friend ran to his car. I thought it was over but he came back with a gun and shot Tom in the stomach."

"Amy, I am so sorry."

"The ambulance came right away but he bled to death before they could get him to the hospital. There wasn't anything I could do."

The location of Amy's pain and Tom's fatal wound matched exactly. The bullet had lacerated the major artery leading to his right leg. She still had nightmares about it. However, the pains did not start until fourteen years after Tom's death. What was the trigger for these attacks?

"Did anything difficult or stressful happen to you just before your pain attacks started?" I asked.

Amy remembered immediately. "I got sick for the first time a few weeks after my Dad died. I went back home for the funeral and I saw the man who shot Tom in a convenience store. He looked right at me but didn't recognize me. It was such a shock to see him because I thought he was still in prison." Seeing him again brought back all the memories and emotions of seeing her brother killed. The pain and vomiting began soon thereafter.

Amy was uncomfortable expressing her emotions verbally and admitted that she probably learned this from her family, which did not communicate well. This explained why Amy's family did not think to warn her that Tom's killer was living in their community again. If verbal outlets for emotions are not available then only physical outlets remain. This might have contributed to her physical symptoms.

Any event associated with intense fear, helplessness or horror can cause stress illness. Surviving an assault, abduction, domestic violence or serious accident, witnessing the unexpected serious injury or death of a loved one or witnessing violence in a military conflict are common examples.

Sometimes the stress illness symptoms occur soon after the event, sometimes not until much later. When symptoms begin after a delay, any of a variety of reminders can be the trigger. Typical reminders include the anniversary of a fearful event, the birthday of a victim of trauma or reading about a similar event. Stress illness caused by trauma can fade in a short time or persist for years. Other symptoms of post-traumatic stress (nightmares, flashbacks, avoidance of reminders) might not occur often or might be much milder than the physical symptoms.

I reassured Amy that with counseling the pain attacks would likely stop. I referred her to a therapist. Six weeks later, Amy returned for her follow-up visit and reported her counseling was going well. Emotions dormant for seventeen years began to surface in therapy. She had no more pain attacks.

TRAUMATIC STRESS: DR. ERDMAN'S STORY

Word of mouth can sometimes be a wonderful thing. Before starting my monthly seminars for patients with stress illness, I publicized the service among my colleagues. Sadly, just one patient came to the first session and I was very disappointed. My wife encouraged me to keep offering the classes and a few more people showed up. Then I began receiving notes from physicians attesting to the benefits their patients were reporting. Attendance increased as the value of the information became more widely known. Before long, two or three dozen patients were coming to each class. Another welcome surprise occurred when the editor of a medical journal telephoned to ask me to write an article about the classes (see Appendix I for the journal reference). Then physicians began attending to learn more about what they had heard from their patients. Sometimes three or four came at once including family practitioners, internists, mental health professionals, gynecologists, pain specialists and an orthopedist (who took care of many people with unexplained back pain).

One of these doctors was Vicky Erdman, a family practitioner in Portland who had cared for a wide variety of patients in clinics all over the country. A week after hearing the seminar she sent me a note that began: "You have completely changed the way I think about patient care." To explain what she meant, Dr. Erdman shared the following story.

Scott was still in his forties, never smoked and had normal cholesterol and excellent blood pressure. However, for three years he had chest pains about once each month that strongly suggested he had heart disease. Tests failed to uncover a cause for the pain (his heart was normal) and various treatments failed to give him any relief. Dr. Erdman was the fourth doctor to try to solve this mystery and she saw him for the first time a few days after she attended the stress illness seminar.

As she talked to him about the five types of stress, he had no difficulty recalling the death of his uncle Walter. It is an old story in the Pacific Northwest. Scott and Walter were out on the river in a drifting rowboat filled with fishing tackle and beer. It was a hot day and their uncomfortable flotation vests soon came off. Walter decided to cool off with a dip over the side into water that originated primarily from a melting glacier. He let go of the gunwale, the current carried him a few yards away and then he began to struggle. Before Scott could even get the boat pointed in the right direction, Walter slipped under the surface and never came up. Now three years later, Scott was still having nightmares several times per month.

Dr. Erdman quickly established the drowning took place only six weeks before Scott's first attack of chest pain. She also learned the first attack occurred while Scott was preparing the boat for his first fishing trip after Walter's death. Several other attacks occurred while Scott was working on the boat and he never managed to get it back on the water. After Dr. Erdman established this connection, Scott began remembering other events that occurred shortly before an attack of chest pain: being invited to go fishing, reading about a drowning in the newspaper and walking down to the river's bank at a picnic.

Dr. Erdman arranged for Scott to see a mental health therapist with experience in post-traumatic stress. Scott responded very well to this treatment and soon his chest pain and nightmares were gone. I am sure it took time before he could fish on the river again, but at least he was on a path that would someday leave the tragedy behind.

TRAUMATIC STRESS: SANDY

Sandy was a fifty-eight-year-old homemaker from Washington who had become the despair of the cardiology department. For eighteen months, she suffered from chest pain attacks that persisted despite a variety of treatments. Her pain began during a trip to Arizona to attend a convention with her husband. After arriving in Phoenix, she woke with a gnawing pain behind her breastbone. She had never had heart trouble, exercised regularly and did not smoke, but her husband took no chances and brought her to the emergency room. The electrocardiogram and blood tests were normal and her pain vanished in a few hours. She returned to Washington with a recommendation from the emergency room physician to have further testing.

A treadmill exercise test showed no heart trouble. This was reassuring, but then the pain began occurring almost every week. It was always in the same location with the same gnawing quality. It came on randomly without any relationship to exercise or meals. It would last from one to several hours and she needed narcotic tablets for relief.

Sandy underwent another treadmill test with the addition of a radioactive tracer. Then she had an ultrasound echo study and finally an angiogram with x-ray dye infused into the heart muscle circulation. None of these showed any problems. She received prescriptions for a number of medicines to treat either poor circulation in the heart muscle or heartburn (in case stomach acid was responsible). Her pain continued unchanged.

We talked about the ability of stress to produce illness and began discussing the five different types. There were no significant sources of stress in her life at that time. Her husband had been ill, but now felt well and was happy in his work. She had no symptoms of depression. There had been no traumatic events in her life at the time the symptoms began.

Sandy and I began talking about her childhood. She and her mother had never been close. Sandy could not recall any abuse, but the general level of emotional support had never been good. Her mother often seemed bitter and Sandy, always eager to please, remembered few smiles or hugs. She talked about her mother for several minutes. Then she finished answering a question and paused, appearing to have more to say. I waited.

After a while, she told me her mother died about three years before. Her mother had lived near Phoenix. While going through her mother's effects after the funeral, Sandy came across a letter in the family Bible. Sandy's mother had written the letter and addressed it to Sandy. It contained a list of "Ten Reasons Why I Hate You." Sandy finished reading, tore the letter to shreds and tried to forget she had ever seen it.

A year and a half later, her husband's convention brought her back to Arizona for the first time since her mother's death. The convention happened to be in Phoenix. The familiar surroundings brought back the memory of the letter. Sandy's emotions had been so strong — and the outlets for them so few — that chest pains were the result.

"So what should I do now?" she asked.

"Write her a reply!" I said. "Put down *your* strongest thoughts and feelings." Communicating emotions in words often means those feelings no longer need expression as physical pain. Writing the words often works better for this purpose than speaking them. Writing has an almost magical ability to help us express ideas we might not fully comprehend otherwise. The fact that her mother was not alive to read Sandy's response was not important. Most of my patients who write letters expressing feelings to their living parents choose not to mail them.

This plan worked well. Writing helped Sandy understand many subtle ways her mother pressured her over the years. The letter in the Bible was just the last and most obvious form of emotional abuse. Once Sandy understood this, she felt relieved of a lifelong burden and her chest pains did not return.

TRAUMATIC STRESS: CHANG

Thirteen-year-old Maya woke up from dreaming that something terrible was going to happen to her father. Maya told her nine-year-old brother Chang about her nightmare and her fears for their father's safety. Later that morning, just before Dad took Chang on a short drive to visit a friend, Maya told Chang to be sure and protect his father that day.

Chang, now twenty-eight, told me the tragic story. "I was playing with my friends behind their house. Then I heard an ambulance siren in the distance. I didn't think anything of it at first but it kept getting louder. Then I remembered it was about time for my father to be picking me up. I got scared, because I remembered what Maya had said."

"What happened next, Chang?"

"I ran to the front of the house. I could see our car at the far end of the street. It was all banged up. I could see them loading my father into the ambulance. I raced down the street but by the time I got there the ambulance was driving away."

"How serious was your father's injury?" I asked.

"His neck was broken. I didn't find that out until later. At the accident, I asked a police officer if my Dad was okay and she told me he just had a "stiff neck," that he would probably be home for dinner. But the ambulance had its lights flashing and the siren was on so I was worried."

Chang's father did not make it home for dinner for nearly eight months. The auto accident left him permanently paralyzed with only limited use of his arms. The first time Chang saw him after the accident was at a rehabilitation center. There was a steel "halo" screwed into his skull and he was strapped into a rotatable bed to prevent pressure sores. He had lost a significant amount of weight, changing the appearance of his face so much that his son had trouble recognizing him. Chang felt completely responsible for not protecting his father after Maya's warning. His guilt was overwhelming.

When his dad finally returned home, Chang devoted himself to caring for him. His mother got a job to support the family and Maya was busy being a teenager. The family was grateful for Chang's devotion though ignorant of the powerful underlying motivation. As he grew older, Chang had problems in school, developed depression and anxiety, began smoking cigarettes and used cocaine periodically.

When I met Chang, he was still living at home and caring for his father nearly twenty years after the accident. He had only recently revealed his sense of responsibility. Chang stopped using drugs and alcohol about three years before. Without those substances to numb his emotional pain, he began having abdominal cramps that grew steadily more severe. Chang's pain was located throughout his abdomen, most often occurring in the evening and early morning hours and had not improved despite a large number of medications. Even two narcotic tablets every six hours failed to provide complete relief. Removal of his gallbladder also did not help even though he had gallstones. Several diagnostic tests were normal. Not one of his many doctors had probed enough to find Chang's heavy emotional burden.

I knew relieving Chang's pain would depend on finding a way to reduce his guilt. We spoke at length of the exact circumstances of his father's accident. We discussed how Chang had been on the other side of his friend's home when it occurred. I pointed out that a neighbor, who witnessed the accident, was much closer to his father at the time, but still unable to prevent the injury. I explained to Chang that because he had not learned the truth about the accident's seriousness until much later, there had been no chance to talk about his feelings at the time. I was also able to help Chang realize that his family's dramatic change in circumstances blinded them to the emotions he was feeling.

Chang had a niece and nephew, now about eight or nine years of age. I asked him to imagine them in his place on the day of the accident and ask if they could have changed the outcome. I told him I heard no evidence that anyone could have prevented his father's tragedy. I asked him to consider how much the guilt had affected his self-image and behavior. I suggested he write a letter to himself as a nine-year-old that would offer forgiveness. I answered his questions, brought his mother into the examination room and then left to arrange referral to a therapist.

When I returned, his mother asked to speak to me alone, saying Chang had explained my diagnosis. He cried through much of their discussion. This was unusual for him, since he usually kept emotions to himself. His mother was hopeful this indicated real change for him.

Chang began seeing the therapist and made steady progress. Before too long, his pain began to fade. Chang moved into an apartment and began, for the first time, to plan a future for himself.

TRAUMATIC STRESS: KANESHA

Kanesha's gallbladder scan was strikingly abnormal. Dr. Navarro, a family practitioner, ordered the scan on thirty-six-year-old Kanesha after three weeks of severe pain in the upper right corner of the abdomen. The gallbladder is right underneath this spot so Dr. Navarro was suspicious this organ was the source of the pain. Even after an ultrasound and blood tests were normal, she ordered the scan as an additional check. The results were a surprise. The radioactive tracer used in the scan flowed into the gallbladder normally, but also appeared to flow into the space between the stomach and the liver. This was outside the gallbladder and suggested the possibility of a leak from the gallbladder or one of the attached ducts. Kanesha might need surgery if this were the case. To find the exact location of the leak, a special x-ray procedure was necessary. I had Kanesha come to the hospital right away.

Kanesha appeared anxious, but not nearly as ill as I had expected. She was dressed in T-shirt and jeans, was about a hundred pounds overweight and wore her hair in a ponytail. Kanesha lived with her mother and worked as an accountant for an auto dealer.

Her physical examination was not consistent with a leaking gallbladder. She had pain and tenderness only in one spot next to the ribs. A leak would produce symptoms across much of her upper abdomen, not just this small area. A leak might also cause fever and should produce several abnormal blood tests and an abnormal ultrasound exam. None of these was present.

I decided not to trust the scan and ordered another one. It looked the same as the first. Dr. Belknap, who performed the second scan, felt sure it was a leak. I asked if there was any other possible explanation for the abnormal image. Dr. Belknap thought for a while. Then he remembered a report in a medical journal of a patient who had tracer in the stomach that happened to be overlapping the liver area. The image in that report looked much like Kanesha's scan. It was unusual, but it could happen. If the tracer was in the stomach and the gallbladder was not leaking, then there was no problem that required treatment. This seemed to be the best explanation for the abnormal scan.

This is an example of what doctors call a false positive test, which is a common problem in stress illness patients. When a diagnostic test (of any type) shows something wrong in a normal area, then the patient usually needs still more testing to prove the first test was wrong. When this happens, the falsely positive test raises hope or fear about a diagnosis, which is then reversed after more studies that could be risky, uncomfortable or expensive. I was convinced Kanesha's scan was a false positive. However, if there was no leak and the rest of her tests were normal, what was causing her pain?

I began asking about sources of stress in her life. Kanesha lived with and cared for her diabetic mother, who was beginning to suffer medical complications. This was not only hard work, but mom criticized Kanesha loudly and often. Kanesha's mother had behaved this way toward all of her children almost from their birth. Nothing the children did was ever good enough for Kanesha's mother. Though she never hit her children, the verbal abuse was just as damaging to their self-esteem.

I asked Kanesha if all the criticism could have become too much to bear. She did not think so. The abuse had been going on for years and Kanesha felt she was "used to it." She could not recall any particular criticism at the time the pain began that was worse or different. "Mom is just Mom, and I do the best I can with her," she said.

She did have some symptoms of depression including significant fatigue, difficulty sleeping and an appetite that was not the best. However, these symptoms had not changed recently and she had no anxiety problems. After nearly an hour, I had covered her symptoms, her childhood, her present day issues, her depression and her mother. Nothing connected clearly to the sudden onset of pain.

"Have you ever experienced any severe traumas in your life?" was my next question. She turned away and stared at the wall. She had been rocking back and forth holding the painful area of her abdomen in her right hand. After my question, she stopped rocking.

"Believe it or not, twelve years ago I was pretty cute," she began. One night I stepped outside a dance club for a smoke and three guys grabbed me..." and here she paused and took a few breaths. "They slapped duct tape on my mouth, threw me into a pickup and put a knife to my throat. They took me to the woods, did their thing and left me there. I was just glad they didn't kill me."

She got medical attention and then tried to forget the rape ever happened. During the next two years, she gained a hundred pounds without knowing why or how. It was suddenly more comfortable for her to be unattractive to men and the extra weight served that purpose.

From the expression on Kanesha's face, I knew this was still a highly emotional episode for her. However, that alone was not enough to be certain the trauma was responsible for her symptoms. I needed to find a link between the assault twelve years ago and the start of her abdominal pain three weeks ago. When I asked her if she could think of such a connection, she knew the answer immediately. On the day before her pain started, she walked into a therapist's office for the first time. She wanted help because the memories of the assault were still bothering her and the nightmares were starting to return.

"The therapist asked me to close my eyes and take myself back to that night. A minute later, I vomited all over his carpet. It happened so fast I couldn't even grab his wastebasket." When she woke up the following morning, the pain began. It was clear to both of us this timing was not a coincidence.

Before I could ask another question, her pain vanished. She did not seem half as surprised as I was at this. She started rubbing the formerly tender spot and confirmed that the pain had simply stopped. This was the first time in three weeks she had been free of pain. I told her we had found the cause of her problem and canceled the special x-ray. Then I recommended that she return to the therapist. As she thought about this, the pain began to come back, though it was now much milder.

I was in touch with her by phone several times over the following six months. Her pain continued to come and go, often related to how difficult her therapy sessions were, but at other times without an obvious trigger. Each time I spoke with her the pain was less. She made excellent progress with the therapist. She never developed any problems with her gallbladder.

TREATMENT FOR TRAUMATIC STRESS

Soldiers returning from the trenches in World War I often suffered from post-traumatic stress. Prevailing medical opinion at the time attributed the symptoms to concussive brain damage from exploding shells. This gave rise to the label "shell shock." Treatment based on this concept had limited value. Today, experienced mental health therapists understand that post-traumatic stress can have many causes including violence from an intimate partner, a motor vehicle accident, an assault or witnessing an event that causes intense fear or horror. Modern treatment is usually successful in managing this condition. A list of the symptoms of post-traumatic stress disorder is in the box.

> ### The Symptoms of Post-Traumatic Stress
>
> - Distressing memories that come back whether you want them to or not
> - Nightmares and flashbacks where you might feel you are reliving the trauma
> - Strong reactions to anything that triggers memories of the trauma
> - Taking steps to avoid reminders of the trauma
> - Feeling keyed up or anxiously watchful much of the time which can interfere with sleep
> - Difficulty experiencing emotions
> - Feeling detached from the world
> - Irritability or outbursts of anger

In some patients with post-traumatic stress, the physical symptoms of stress illness bring them to the doctor. In these cases, revealing the mental and emotional problems caused by the trauma requires specific questioning. Whether the symptoms are physical or emotional or both, a mental health therapist with experience in managing post-traumatic stress is the best resource.

The first task in treatment is to ensure personal safety. If the patient is not safe (because of ongoing violence from an intimate partner, for example), the trauma will limit the benefit of any form of treatment. A social worker, family therapist or other experienced professional can be helpful in making the transition to a safe environment. In some cases, staying at a safe house or shelter could be essential to ensure physical safety.

After securing personal safety, counseling is the next step. A discussion of the common symptoms that follow a traumatic event can help a survivor better comprehend their situation. Knowing that the distressing symptoms described above are normal reactions is reassuring. Post-trauma support groups can be a valuable source of further education.

Medication can help, though it might require several weeks to achieve full benefit. Medicines developed to treat depression have proven to be useful in controlling post-trauma symptoms. In particular, antidepressants that enhance serotonin levels in the brain such as fluoxetine and sertraline are quite effective. Trazodone is another antidepressant useful for post-trauma symptoms, especially for those with insomnia or nightmares. New medicines that might be helpful appear on the market regularly.

A medicine called clonidine lowers blood pressure. In post-traumatic stress, it can help by modifying signals from the stress response center in the brain. It can reduce high levels of vigilance, anger outbursts, jumpiness and nightmares.

If symptoms persist despite education and medication, then psychotherapy is usually necessary. A variety of beneficial techniques is available, including relaxation techniques such as the one described in the chapter on treating current stress. Individual counseling, group therapy, family therapy and desensitization treatment are also used. The latter method emphasizes relaxation technique while exposing the patient to limited reminders of the trauma in a controlled and supportive environment. Gradually, tolerance for increasingly difficult reminders is developed. Post-traumatic stress disorder responds well to treatment. As the post-trauma symptoms improve, the physical symptoms of stress illness tend to improve as well.

CHAPTER 6
DEPRESSION

*When depression is stigmatized as illness and weakness,
a double bind is created: If we admit to depression, we
will be stigmatized by others; if we feel it but do not
admit it, we stigmatize ourselves, internalizing the
social judgment.... The only remaining choice may be
truly sick behavior: to experience no emotion at all.*

– Lesley Hazelton

DEPRESSION: SAM

SAM WAS A SIXTY-ONE-YEAR-OLD MECHANICAL ENGINEER WHO HAD SEEN MORE
doctors in the last ten weeks than he usually did in ten years. In the middle
of an unusually wet winter, he gradually became aware he did not feel quite
right. He found his symptoms difficult to put into words. To some of his
physicians he would say he was nauseated. To others that he just did not feel
himself. On other occasions, he would point to his abdomen as the source of
an abnormal sensation or an ache. Over three to four months he lost fifteen
pounds from his already lean frame. His doctor's greatest concern was the
weight loss and he suspected Sam had a cancer or other serious problem.

The diagnostic tests began. Tube after tube of blood, a urine specimen,
ultrasounds, x-rays, scans and internal video exams were done, all of them
entirely normal. This was reassuring, but Sam felt even worse after the two
months of testing. His family wondered if an MRI (magnetic resonance imaging) test might be the answer.

In reviewing his symptoms, I noticed his difficulty describing exactly what
was wrong. Depression often produces a vague, difficult to describe feeling of
being unwell. Sam told me he did not feel depressed but he did feel fatigued
and his appetite was off. In addition, he often awoke at 3:00 or 4:00 AM and

was unable to return to sleep. None of his doctors had asked him about these common symptoms of depression because they focused on finding a visible cause of his illness.

"Sam, there is a good chance that you are suffering from an imbalance of neurotransmitters in your brain," I told him.

"How can you tell that?" he asked.

"We don't have any way to measure neurotransmitters. But an imbalance can cause all the symptoms you have and we haven't found anything else wrong with you," I replied.

"So what do we do?"

"I would like to prescribe a medication that is designed to percolate through the nervous system and correct any imbalances that are present. Medicines that do this were invented to treat depression because depression is caused by the same kind of chemical imbalance. But if you don't feel depressed they can still help the other symptoms you have."

"Is it addictive?" he asked.

"Antidepressants are not addictive, tranquilizing or mind-altering. They work by restoring a compound that the body needs to function normally. The benefit is similar to giving insulin to a diabetic. Without neurotransmitters, your brain is like an automobile with water in the gas tank. The machine is fine, but the fuel is wrong."

"Won't this medicine just be treating the symptoms and covering up the real problem?" he wondered.

"This medicine treats the real underlying problem. If I'm wrong about your diagnosis the medicine won't help you at all. If I'm right you should feel better in two to six weeks. In that sense, taking this medicine is like a diagnostic test as well as a treatment."

"At this point I'm about ready to try anything. This is the first hope I've had in months."

Within two weeks of beginning treatment, he reported his problems were 50 percent improved. After a month, all the stomach symptoms stopped and he was rapidly regaining weight. In addition, Sam's energy returned, he could sleep through the night and he enjoyed eating again. No further diagnostic tests were needed.

DEPRESSION: LAURA

Except for one enormous secret, Laura would have fit any political pollster's definition of a soccer mom. She was thirty-seven, married, worked part-time in a bookstore and ferried her son and daughter to their athletic practices and games year-round. For the last three years, though, she had seen her doctor almost every month for a variety of symptoms that never had a confirmed diagnosis and always got better with simple treatments. She was in my office because her latest symptom — abdominal pains — refused to go away. Several diagnostic tests were normal.

She did not appear the least bit depressed. She smiled, joked, laughed and seemed to have all the energy needed to manage her many responsibilities. However, on direct questioning it turned out she was waking in the early hours of the morning, her energy level was a fraction of where it had been five years before and her enthusiasm for life had been lacking for some time. She found herself pushing hard to make it through each day and collapsing after dinner. When I asked her if she felt depressed, she looked shocked, as if I had guessed a carefully guarded secret.

Laura was quick to admit she felt depressed, but had kept this from her husband, her co-workers and even her family doctor. Then she told me about the garden hose.

"I bought it three years ago," she began. This was just at the time when her frequent visits to her doctor had begun. "I put it in the trunk of my car. I was going to run exhaust from the tailpipe into the car to kill myself."

"What kept you from going through with it?" I asked.

"I was just waiting for one more thing to go wrong."

Not everyone improves with the first antidepressant they are prescribed, but fortunately for Laura, the benefits were dramatic. When she returned after six weeks for her follow-up visit, she told me she was amazed at how different she felt. Her depressed mood lifted, she could sleep through the night and her zest for life returned. She used the hose only to water her garden.

DEPRESSION: LISA

Until recently, nothing could stop Lisa from making exquisite jewelry, which she sold all over the Northwest. She was fifty-four and came to my office from her cabin on the Oregon coast wearing many of her creations. She had been healthy until twenty months earlier when she suddenly felt pain in her rectum and buttock area. She also noticed it went down the side of her right thigh at times. The pain was present twenty-four hours a day and was unrelated to her bowel movements.

Beyond this, Lisa could only describe the symptoms in vague terms. I tried to pin her down to specifics. Was the pain near the surface or deep inside? Was it burning, sharp, dull, aching or throbbing? Which area had the most intense pain? Was there anything that made it worse or better? She was not sure about any of these.

Lisa's difficulty describing the symptoms was a clue they might be stress-related. So was the fact that three doctors, a CAT scan and a video exam of her large intestine failed to find any problems. She also used phrases like "I'm at the end of my rope," "I'm all worn out" and "The pain keeps me from wanting to go anywhere." Comments like these are frequent in people with depression. At times, tears were visible in her eyes and she admitted to crying at home, "sometimes over just a TV commercial."

She had several other symptoms consistent with depression. She woke in the early morning three or four nights a week and was unable to return to sleep. She also felt tired most of the time, to the point that her energy for working on jewelry "just isn't there any more." She felt down more days than not. I was disappointed to learn that none of her other doctors had asked about these problems.

We had a long discussion about the ability of depression to cause illness. Suddenly, Lisa remembered an incident that occurred fifty years ago.

"I just remembered the strangest thing. I don't know why I didn't think of it before," she began. "When I was four years old, my older brother kicked me right in the tailbone. For days, I couldn't sit down or even walk normally. I think it was the same pain I am having now."

I can only speculate about this coincidence. We assume that symptoms in stress illness result from nerve signals traveling from the stress response center to the affected area(s) of the body. Usually there is no obvious reason symptoms occur at one site instead of another. However, in Lisa the pain nerve pathway to her buttock might have retained an effect from the childhood injury that caused it to be re-used when she developed depression. I observed a similar phenomenon in a patient several years after an appendectomy. Another patient who experienced back pain for a year after a motor vehicle accident in 1973 developed stress illness symptoms in the same location in 1993.

Lisa had concluded she was beyond help. Fortunately, with antidepressant medication she experienced dramatic relief from her pain and her depression symptoms. She soon returned to her jewelry workshop as if she had never left it.

DEPRESSION: DIANE

Diane was disgusted with the quality of her medical care. After over a year of pain in her abdomen, a lump in her throat, soreness in her lower left leg, a noticeable increase in the frequency of her migraines, constant nausea and frequent constipation it seemed like all her many doctors simply stopped listening. Her chart showed a long list of medical problems although depression was not among them. "I'm exhausted and frustrated, but I'm not depressed," she said through her tears.

However, it was a rare night when she slept for longer than two hours at a time. Her appetite was gone. Her trips to the community pool had fallen from three or four each week to zero. Sexual activity with her husband had declined considerably and she found herself crying more than she ever had in her life.

This also was not the first time she suffered these symptoms. As a child, she struggled constantly with physical and sexual abuse from as far back as she could remember. When she was five years old, she went to the medicine cabinet, found a bottle with a poison symbol on it, poured the contents into a bowl of cereal and started eating with every intention of killing herself. Fortunately, the bottle was nearly empty, the cereal diluted the drug and the taste was so bad she could not finish eating it. Her parents treated this as a mere accident.

This incident took place thirty years ago. I can't be sure what was in her mind back then, but Diane had no doubt she understood what she was doing and meant to end her life. Remarkably, it was the only suicide attempt of her life. I still struggle to understand how she found the courage and strength to survive thirteen more years of abuse before she could finally leave her home. Being able to help people who are so determined and who have endured so much is one of the many rewards of caring for people with stress illness.

I was able to persuade Diane that it was possible to suffer from the disease depression without the symptom of feeling depressed. I pointed out that many depression sufferers feel exhaustion or frustration instead. With medication and regular counseling from a therapist, Diane's many symptoms improved considerably in the next several months.

TREATMENT OF DEPRESSION

Depression can be a subtle disease, causing physical symptoms and making life more difficult to cope with even in people who do not look depressed. A simplified discussion of the physiology of depression will provide a convenient way to understand its diagnosis and treatment.

Nerve cells in the brain and body do not touch each other, so they cannot send signals electrically like the wires in your home. Instead, when one nerve cell needs to communicate with another, it uses a chemical messenger called a neurotransmitter (pronounced, "ner oh tranz mitt er"). If certain neurotransmitter levels are too low, nerve cells cannot communicate normally and depression can result.

What causes this decline in chemical supply? In some people, the nervous system simply is not manufacturing enough. People with this problem often tell me they have no reason to feel depressed because their lives are going well. I explain that their illness is similar to diabetes where the body does not have enough insulin. If your nervous system is not making enough neurotransmitters, you can develop depression even if your life is wonderful otherwise. In other people, depression seems to develop after many years of suffering from stress. In these situations, stress might be reducing the levels of neurotransmitters. We cannot measure your neurotransmitters directly, but we suspect they are below normal if you develop the symptoms of depression. There is a list of these in the box.

The Symptoms of Depression

- Feeling depressed, down or hopeless

- Crying frequently for no obvious reason

- Fatigue

- Believing that life is no longer worth living and that death might be preferable to the emotional suffering (if you feel this way, contact a doctor immediately)

- Difficulty falling asleep or difficulty remaining asleep through the night

- Decreasing enthusiasm for activities previously enjoyed

- Losing interest in food. Weight loss might occur because of reduced eating. Some patients eat more when depressed and might gain weight

- Inability to cope with normal day-to-day stresses

- Having a shorter temper or feeling more irritable

- Feeling worthless or guilty

- Difficulty concentrating

Some depressed people have just a few of these symptoms and others have many. *It is important to recognize that people can have this disorder without feeling particularly depressed.* Any person with several symptoms on the list above is likely suffering from depression. Many patients have difficulty accepting a diagnosis of depression when they do not feel that way. I ask them to think of themselves as having a neurotransmitter imbalance instead.

Depression can become severe enough to produce the physical symptoms of stress illness, even when there are no other significant stresses present. The story of Sam, who described his symptoms in different ways to each doctor, is a good example. Depression can also magnify other stresses and make them more difficult to manage. Those other stresses can then make the depression worse. A vicious cycle can result as depression reduces the ability to cope, which makes other stresses more difficult, which then makes the depression worse. Some of my patients with depression lived in this vicious cycle for so long that even relatively minor physical symptoms seem overwhelming. One woman came to the emergency room, curled up on a bed and began crying softly. She could no longer tolerate her "severe diarrhea," which I learned consisted of just three or four soft movements daily. The diarrhea stopped when her depression was successfully treated.

Another man came in for evaluation of abdominal complaints. His first statement was "I just can't take the wind any more, Doc." As a gastroenterologist, I assumed he was complaining about passing too much intestinal gas. He was actually referring to the noise of the wind blowing around his home. But he had lived in the same windy area for the last fifteen years and only in the last twelve months did this bother him. He also had several other symptoms of depression. After treatment with an antidepressant, those symptoms and his concerns about the wind went away.

Management of depression requires experience and judgment. The first step is evaluation by an experienced professional who can help you decide if your treatment should use medication, counseling or both. These are effective in about 80 percent of cases. We will look at medications first.

Antidepressant medicines (there are many) can be very helpful, especially in more severe depression. Even better, they are not tranquilizers, they are not addictive and they do not create unwanted personality changes. In some people, antidepressant medication alone can relieve symptoms significantly.

Some patients are reluctant to take medication that creates changes in the brain. Remember, though, that the brain is a flesh and blood organ like any other and therefore subject to biochemical dysfunction just like the heart, liver or kidneys. Because antidepressant medication works by correcting these abnormalities, this treatment is similar to a diabetic patient taking insulin. In diabetes, we try to improve health by correcting a deficiency of the essential protein insulin. Antidepressant medication also corrects a deficiency. We do not expect diabetics simply to "snap out of" their disease with will power. I don't expect people to overcome depression this way either.

It is important to understand that antidepressants need a few weeks to create a noticeable change and four to six weeks to achieve full effectiveness. Patients should also be aware that these medicines differ from one another with respect to their benefits for particular symptoms. Doctors experienced with antidepressants can choose a drug that will match a person's particular needs. For example, some antidepressants are better than others for helping you sleep. Others can give you more energy during the day or will be more effective if you also experience anxiety. If one medicine is not helpful, another could work better and some trial and error in this process is common. After you identify a beneficial medicine, continuing it for at least nine to twelve months will significantly reduce the risk of a relapse. Some people need medication only once in their lives. They can taper the dose and then stop completely. Other people, especially those with recurring episodes of depression, require treatment intermittently or indefinitely. Advice from a qualified doctor is essential in making decisions about the duration of treatment.

Antidepressants can cause side effects. Just as it is common to need trial and error to find a medicine with the best results for symptoms, it is also common to need a few tries before finding a drug with a minimum of side effects. Most of the time, the benefits of these medicines far outweigh their problems. Side effects of some of these medicines are dry mouth, constipation, weight gain, difficulty with having a sexual climax and increased anxiety or agitation. If side effects are a problem, good alternative medication is available for most patients.

St. John's wort is an herbal remedy for depression that is more effective than placebo for mild chemical imbalance. Side effects are uncommon. However, studies have reported interference between St. John's wort and medications used for:

- Treating HIV infection (the virus that causes AIDS)
- Slowing blood coagulation ("blood thinner" medicines)
- Preventing rejection of heart transplants
- Birth control

You should not combine St. John's wort with other antidepressants such as fluoxetine and similar drugs. A major study of St. John's wort published in the *Journal of the American Medical Association* in April of 2001 found no benefit in moderate or major depression. Other herbal remedies such as Valerian and Kavakava also do not have evidence of benefit in this condition.

Though many primary care doctors are skilled in prescribing these medicines, a mental health professional can be a valuable resource by providing counseling or extra assistance in prescribing. The combination of medication and counseling is often more effective than either alone. The involvement of a mental health professional is particularly valuable for those who:

- Have suicidal thoughts or plans (contact a health professional immediately if you have this)
- Have tried one or two medications and have not improved
- Require two or more medicines simultaneously
- Have a history of manic episodes
- Have auditory or visual hallucinations

Mental health counseling also has an important role in treatment because medication alone will not improve life stresses that are contributing to the depression. For example, if problems in a marriage or at work are significant, a tablet will not change them. For many patients counseling alone is adequate treatment, making medication unnecessary.

A counselor will often begin by helping clients understand the many distressing symptoms depression can cause and that effective treatment is available. This provides reassurance and hope. A counselor can then provide perspective on the individual's strengths, weaknesses, expectations, and goals and the impressions of those who know them. Depression can distort perception of these. For example, some depressed people are overly self-critical or have limited goals for the future.

Counseling can help assess the relative magnitude of problems in life. This can lead to constructive plans for solving these dilemmas. A counselor can also explore links between depression and mistreatment in childhood. This can improve understanding of the roots of the illness. For all these reasons, an experienced therapist can be essential for the best outcome.

CHAPTER 7
ANXIETY DISORDERS

If a person lost would conclude that after all he is not lost, he is not beside himself, but standing in his own old shoes on the very spot where he is, and that for the time being he will live there; but the places that have known him, they are lost,—how much anxiety and danger would vanish.

– Henry David Thoreau

ANXIETY: BRENNA

BRENNA WAS EMBARRASSED DURING EVERY ONE OF HER HIGH SCHOOL SOCCER games, but not because of how she played. She was not the star of the team, but she made varsity as a sophomore and now, as a junior, started every game in the key position of center midfielder. Unfortunately, as soon as the whistle blew for half-time, she would race for the locker room because of diarrhea. This began every fall during soccer season and was getting worse every year. Tests done by her family doctor were normal.

The pattern of her diarrhea was unusual. In addition to her symptoms at half-time, Brenna had her worst problems in the mornings on Tuesdays and Thursdays and she took up to a half dozen antidiarrhea tablets within a few hours on those days. Her symptoms became so severe she would avoid eating on the bad days and she lost over ten pounds. Brenna's condition was much better on weekends when she sometimes took no antidiarrhea medication at all. There was no difference in her diet on any day of the week except for eating less on the bad days.

It turned out that her school played all girls' soccer games on Tuesdays and Thursdays. She admitted to feeling extremely tense about these games. At times, she developed shortness of breath and a tingling sensation in her fingers and toes that probably resulted from rapid deep breathing (hyperventilation). All this sounded quite a bit like an anxiety disorder, specifically the one known as generalized anxiety disorder. It was unlikely that diarrhea caused by inflamed or infected bowels or any other cause would vary so enormously depending on the day of the week. I prescribed an anti-anxiety medication called paroxetine and, within two weeks, she amazed her teammates by playing complete games without needing a bathroom break. She no longer needed any medicine for diarrhea and ate a normal diet.

The anxiety disorders are found in nearly one of every five people who visit a primary care physician. Anxiety disorders cause people to feel nervous, anxious, on edge or afraid or to have trouble relaxing more days than not and out of proportion to any reason for those feelings to be present. Often no reason for those feelings is apparent. In many people, the anxiety disorders also cause symptoms in the body and these can be what bring the sufferer to medical attention. Doctors sometimes focus on the physical symptoms so much that they fail to consider the correct diagnosis of an anxiety disorder.

Symptoms of Generalized Anxiety Disorder

Persistent, excessive anxiety or worry about common events or activities occurring more days than not for at least six months. Worry can focus on personal, family, financial, job or security issues. The degree of anxiety is greater than seems reasonable for the given circumstances, is difficult to control and can interfere with performing usual tasks.

Other associated symptoms can include fatigue, restlessness, difficulty concentrating, irritability and disrupted sleep.

Associated physical symptoms can include muscle tension, sweats, cold hands or feet, difficulty swallowing, nausea, abdominal discomfort and change in bowel habit.

ANXIETY: SARAH

For several years, twenty-nine-year-old Sarah had one or two episodes each week of an urgent need to have a bowel movement coupled with a strong fear of not being near enough to a bathroom. At first, I had some difficulty getting details from Sarah because her eighteen-month-old son Joshua was with her and created quite a disruption. So I gave him a plastic rectal probe to play with (it was all I could find in the exam room and was brand new, of course). He was so fascinated I told Sarah he would probably grow up to become a proctologist.

Along with her urgent bowel movements, she also had a tingling sensation throughout her body (probably caused by hyperventilation) and a pounding heartbeat. She became extremely reluctant to leave her home unless she was sure a convenient toilet would be available. As long as she was at home, she never had an attack but even while at home she admitted to worrying excessively about many aspects of her life.

Like Brenna, Sarah had generalized anxiety disorder. Prescription of the same anti-anxiety medication Brenna received led to considerable improvement. The attacks became much less frequent and she was able to leave her home far more easily though some of her fear persisted. The tense environment in Sarah's childhood home probably contributed to her symptoms although many patients with anxiety disorders have no obvious cause for their problem. A mental health counselor treated her for a number of months and she made excellent progress. I am not sure about Joshua's current career plans, but our nurses enjoyed seeing him leave the office proudly clutching the probe.

ANXIETY: GERI

Geri was a plump woman in her thirties who was not convinced she needed to see me. She cancelled a few appointments for personal reasons and by the time we met, her stomach had felt normal for nearly three months. Prior to that, she suffered three episodes of severe pain throughout her abdomen lasting up to twelve hours. These occurred a few weeks apart and the emergency room evaluations were normal.

Fortunately, Geri had noticed an important coincidence. All three episodes of pain began when she was in the presence of a large number of people. The first was a birthday party for a friend, the second an Independence Day barbecue at her husband's lodge and the third at a restaurant with her husband and four other couples. For as long as Geri could remember, being around other people had caused her to feel "stress" by which she meant a high level of worry not justified by the circumstances. Usually this resulted in tightening of the muscles around her neck and shoulders. She would also find herself wondering if other people were making judgments about her appearance or behavior and she had an unreasonable fear of being embarrassed. (It was not surprising to learn that Geri's job was on the night shift at a printing press. She liked this shift because "there was no one else around." She also shopped for groceries late at night to avoid crowds.)

When getting out of bed to begin her day she had no muscle tightness. However, as soon as she left the house the tightness began. In the last year, the muscle tightening had grown steadily worse. After her three attacks of abdominal pain, she decided never to go out to dinner with more than one other couple at a time. She avoided parties completely.

Geri had social anxiety disorder. I prescribed medication that provided substantial relief for her "stress" and her muscle tightening. I also referred her to a counselor and gradually she increased the number of people with whom she could be comfortable.

Symptoms of Social Anxiety Disorder

Excessive anxiety and self-consciousness regularly triggered by one or more types of social situations. The individual fears personal embarrassment or judgment by others. These problems can interfere with performing usual tasks, with social activities and with relationships. Sufferers recognize that their fears are unreasonable but are unable to overcome them.

Symptoms might occur only in particular social circumstances (public speaking, eating with others, meeting someone new) or can occur whenever the individual is around other people.

Stress illness symptoms that commonly accompany social anxiety include blushing, sweating, trembling, nausea, diarrhea and difficulty speaking, any of which can compound the person's embarrassment and worry about being judged.

ANXIETY: JOE

Joe, a plumber, owned "one of the most beautiful motorcycles ever made." He loved to ride six or eight hours at a time to destinations around the Pacific

Northwest. A year before our first encounter he was enjoying a fly-fishing trip in Idaho when he suddenly developed severe chest pain and shortness of breath. His friends rushed him to the hospital, but by the time he arrived, he was feeling better. He stayed overnight, but all the tests were negative.

He had a treadmill test of his heart done when he returned home to Washington. This was normal, which was reassuring evidence that his heart was not diseased. He felt well for several weeks, but then another attack hit — every bit as severe as the first. This led to an angiogram, which showed no obstruction of the flow of blood to his heart, followed by tests for adrenaline-producing tumors, abnormal electrical rhythms of the heart and thyroid disease. All were normal. Because both episodes had occurred during motorcycle trips, Joe began cutting back on how far he traveled.

Other conditions that might explain Joe's symptoms included muscle spasm of his esophagus or severe heartburn. Heartburn results from stomach acid reaching the esophagus, a condition called acid reflux. His family practice physician prescribed a strong medicine for suppressing stomach acid, which did nothing for his attacks.

Before our first appointment, he called from Seattle to report another attack. In the course of describing the symptoms he said, "I was really afraid I was dying, Doc." People having a panic attack often feel that way so I asked him if he noticed numbness or tingling in his hands, feet or lips. This symptom can result from hyperventilation that often accompanies panic attacks. It turned out his hands always tingled during his attacks, but he had not thought to mention it to his other doctors. The doctors had not asked him because they focused on his heart and did not consider the possibility that he was having panic attacks. Numbness and tingling would also be unusual if he had acid reflux or muscle spasm of the esophagus so I became more confident that panic attacks were responsible for Joe's symptoms.

After a detailed discussion, Joe agreed to try a dose of a rapidly acting anti-anxiety medicine (related to valium) as a diagnostic test. He was to take the tablet as soon as he had any indication another attack was starting. This medicine would not help if some other disease caused his episodes. A few weeks later, the opportunity to use it occurred and the attack stopped "like turning off a switch, Doc." I referred Joe to our mental health department for further treatment of his panic disorder and he has done well ever since.

Symptoms of Panic Disorder

Recurring panic attacks not caused by disease, medication, illegal drugs, post-traumatic stress or phobias. A panic attack consists of a limited period of sudden, intense fear that peaks within ten minutes and has at least four of the following symptoms:

- Pounding heart, often with pain or discomfort in the chest
- Shortness of breath or feeling of choking
- Feeling lightheaded or dizzy
- Fear of losing control, going crazy or dying
- Sweats, chills or flushing
- Trembling
- Numbness or tingling in the hands or feet
- Nausea or abdominal discomfort

Associated with the panic attacks is at least one month of worry that you will have another one, sometimes accompanied by changing your behavior to reduce the number of attacks.

TREATMENT OF THE ANXIETY DISORDERS

In many ways, management of anxiety is analogous to management of depression. Working with a qualified professional is essential. The mainstays of treatment include medication to correct chemical imbalances in the nervous system, mental health counseling or a combination of these. It turns out that the same medications used for depression are often very helpful in relieving anxiety. In particular, the class of antidepressant medications known as SSRIs (which includes fluoxetine, paroxetine and many others) has become the first choice for most patients. As with the treatment of depression, these medicines need several weeks to achieve their maximum benefit. Another similarity to depression treatment is that if the first SSRI medicine is ineffective for a patient, sometimes a different SSRI will prove beneficial.

Another class of medications, with the jaw-mangling name of benzodiazepines (pronounced, "ben zoh dye aze ah peens" or "benzos" for short) can relieve symptoms during the weeks that the SSRIs need to become effective. The benzos can be habit-forming if taken too frequently for too long but they have a role in providing short-term, rapid symptom relief for many patients.

There is a particular form of mental health counseling, called cognitive-behavioral therapy (CBT), which studies have shown to be effective in the anxiety disorders. As you might guess from the name, CBT has two parts. The cognitive part uses counseling to help you change beliefs that lead to worry and fear. In Geri's case, for example, a counselor might help her understand that people are not judging her and point out that she has rarely embarrassed herself in front of others.

The behavioral part of CBT aims to relieve your physical and emotional reactions to anxious situations. To accomplish this, the counselor exposes you to a mild source of fear in a limited, systematic and controlled way. Again using Geri as an example, she might start by shopping for groceries at a time when a few people are likely to be present. If she handles that well, her next attempt might be when even more people are present. She might never be able to shop for food on the day before Thanksgiving but she would likely make steady progress using this technique, possibly with the support of an SSRI medication.

Anxiety disorders can relapse even after successful treatment. If that happens, the relapses usually respond to treatment just as well as the initial episode and sometimes even faster if you learned CBT skills during a previous episode.

FINDING A THERAPIST

Many stress illness patients benefit from counseling by a skilled mental health professional. But how do you find a good one? The best place to start is with your personal physician. Your doctor can help you decide if counseling is right for you. If it is, they can recommend a therapist and possibly prescribe medication to relieve some of your symptoms until you see the therapist. If possible, try to find a mental health counselor who has special training and experience with your particular concern. (For example, experience with CBT is helpful for people with anxiety disorders.) In addition and if needed, they should be able to arrange for you to receive prescription medication. Access to group therapy can be another useful option, particularly for those with social anxiety disorder.

Feel free to contact a mental health professional before beginning treatment with them. Ask them the questions in the box below and, if you do not feel comfortable with the answers, then ask your doctor, a social worker or the mental health department at the nearest medical school for another recommendation. You can do the same if you begin treatment with someone but later feel unable to collaborate with them. (Be aware, however, that you should not stop certain medications abruptly, but rather should taper the dose gradually to avoid withdrawal symptoms. Use your doctor for advice.)

Questions to Ask a Therapist

Begin by explaining why you would like the therapist's help. Then consider asking the following questions.

What is your training and experience with problems like mine?

How do you treat disorders like mine? Would group therapy or CBT be appropriate for me?

Do you prescribe medication or have access to someone who can prescribe?

Can you estimate how long my treatment might take?

How long are the treatment sessions and how often?

Will it be necessary to include family members in therapy?

What are your fees? Are there any adjustments for financial circumstances?

What kinds of health insurance do you accept?

CHAPTER 8
MULTI-FACTORED STRESS ILLNESS

We all enter the world with fairly simple needs: to be protected, to be nurtured, to be loved unconditionally, and to belong.

– Louise Hart

THOUGH MANY CASES OF STRESS ILLNESS RESULT PRIMARILY FROM A SINGLE TYPE OF stress, many other patients suffer from multiple stresses that can interact with each other. The stories in this chapter illustrate a variety of issues including the influence of religious beliefs and problems common in adolescence.

STRESS PAST AND PRESENT: JENNIFER

At first, I could not make any sense of Jennifer's illness. She was a happily married mother of Nathan, a one-year-old boy who recently took his first steps. Jennifer's illness began when she and her husband were at a friend's home for a birthday party. While eating appetizers, Jennifer began to feel a knot in the middle of her stomach. Within half an hour she was in significant pain and felt increasingly nauseated. Jennifer's husband noticed how pale she looked and drove her straight to the hospital. The emergency room ran several tests, but found no abnormalities. After a few hours, Jennifer felt better and was able to return home. By the next morning, the pain was gone.

Over the next few months, the same pain returned several times, though it was never as severe or as long as the first attack. Her doctor ran several more tests, also with normal results. No one asked her about stress. Then Jennifer and her husband went to dinner at a favorite restaurant to celebrate their second anniversary. The mysterious pain struck again, this time beginning before they arrived at the restaurant and even worse than the initial episode. They left for the emergency room before ordering any food. Once again, all the tests were normal and when the pain eased by midnight she returned home. She called her doctor the next day and came to see me after a few more tests gave no answers.

Jennifer was concerned about food allergy or poisoning. I assured her this was unlikely because her two worst attacks had occurred after different foods and her husband usually ate the same food without becoming ill. I also pointed out some of her other attacks were not food-related and she had eaten nothing at the restaurant. After her exam and a review of tests conducted earlier, I began asking her about each of the five different types of stress.

Initially she could not think of any significant current stress in her life. She had no symptoms of depression or anxiety and could not recall any traumatic events. It is a good thing that subconscious stresses strong enough to cause physical symptoms are usually close to the surface. The general conversations I have with patients about stress nearly always bring these issues into the open before long. This is exactly what happened with Jennifer.

"I don't know what made me think of this, but when I was a kid my parents used to fight with each other all the time," Jennifer remembered.

"Do you mean that they would hit each other?" I asked.

"No, not that. It was more they just constantly bickered and usually over nothing."

They divorced when Jennifer was a teenager. The parents argued with Jennifer, too, and this was still occurring since her mother lived nearby. Jennifer always tried to meet her mother's expectations, but her best efforts frequently were not good enough. As a student, if her usually perfect report cards contained a B instead of an A, Jennifer could count on her parents asking about her plans for improvement. Jennifer's frustration and resentment about all this grew over the years. Unfortunately, she could find nothing to change the situation, so she kept her feelings inside. I was not sure how this might relate to her illness, but as Jennifer kept talking, she remembered another example of the problems her mother could cause.

"She told me she would babysit Nathan while my husband and I went to our friend's birthday party. While we were getting dressed she called up and canceled."

"What reason did she give for canceling?" I asked.

"Just because she didn't feel like babysitting that night." Jennifer had to scramble to find a replacement, but kept her frustration to herself. I noticed that her fists clenched as she told this story.

"Then she did the same thing, canceling at the last minute, on our anniversary," said Jennifer. Again, there was a last minute rush to find another sitter. Jennifer quietly thought about this a little longer. Suddenly, she remembered that those were the two nights she had suffered her worst attacks of pain. Jennifer's frustration with her mother pushed her to the point of physical illness on those evenings.

While growing up, Jennifer learned to suppress her feelings about her constantly arguing parents and their criticism of her best efforts. She suppressed her frustration again on the two nights her mother backed out of babysitting. However, on those evenings the feelings were so strong that when she did not express them in words, they were expressed via her body instead. As she continued to review other milder episodes of pain, she remembered that many of them occurred soon after disagreeable interactions with her mother.

Jennifer was a little embarrassed she had not made this connection sooner. However, it is common not to perceive these associations. This is especially true if you learned at an early age how to suppress your frustration. It amazes me, though, how often a simple conversation about stress will help a patient find the hidden sources of their illness.

Jennifer wondered why she had become ill now, since the most severe episodes of stress from her mother had occurred years earlier. Her mother's behavior had not changed. What was different now? Often the difference is improvement in self-esteem. People who feel better about themselves become less tolerant of ill treatment by others. Sometimes a new and positive relationship can make the crucial difference in self-esteem. Jennifer had been married for only two years.

"Is your husband good to you?" I asked.

"He's the best," she replied. He brought her flowers, he helped prepare meals, he told her she was wonderful and he was a good father to their son.

"Then you might have the Good Partner/Bad Illness syndrome," I told her. In Jennifer's case, the origin of this problem was mistreatment early in life that stunted her self-esteem. When her belief in herself improved, she was able to accept a supportive relationship with her husband. His love helped Jennifer recognize she had never deserved such poor treatment from her parents. She became less accepting of her mother's disregard of her feelings. Jennifer's frustration began to grow, but not her ability to express it in words. Instead, her emotions expressed themselves as abdominal pain.

Jennifer needed no treatment other than recognizing the connection to her mother's behavior. Over time, Jennifer learned to put her feelings into words when difficulties arose and to manage her mother with less guilt and resentment. She was able to let go of her sense of obligation to solve her parents' problems. She suffered no further pain attacks.

The stress in the present from Jennifer's mother was probably not enough to cause pain by itself. Magnification of the stress by hidden links to the past was a key factor in Jennifer's illness. A similar connection to the past was part of Deborah's illness.

MULTIPLE STRESSES: DEBORAH

Deborah's gynecologist was increasingly suspicious that his diagnosis was wrong. Deborah was forty, an avid middle-distance runner and mother of two pre-teens. She was articulate and smiled easily though never for very long. Her gynecologist had evaluated her for intermittent attacks of severe pelvic pain. With the pain, Deborah had a vaginal discharge that seemed to improve with antibiotics. He assumed these attacks were due to pelvic inflammatory disease (PID), an infection of the pelvic organs.

The gynecologist was now questioning this diagnosis because tests for infection during each of Deborah's several attacks of pain were all negative. In addition, transmission of PID infection occurs sexually and Deborah was quite certain her husband was faithful. It is most unusual to have repeated attacks of PID unless you are promiscuous or your partner is infected and neither was the case.

The gynecologist referred Deborah to me to see if her pain might be from an intestinal or stress problem. I found she had no intestinal symptoms and her physical examination was entirely normal. The interview then focused on sources of stress in Deborah's life. She told me her marriage was happy, her children were healthy and she enjoyed her work as a full-time art teacher. On weekends, she was active in volunteer organizations. She did not feel at all depressed, but did have some difficulty sleeping and often felt fatigued.

"Were you under any stress as a child?" I asked. Deborah's parents divorced when she was in pre-school. The few times she saw her father after the divorce, he had great difficulty providing emotional support. Her mother remarried when Deborah reached middle school, but the stepfather never showed much interest in Deborah.

"My mother also had very high standards," she continued. "I used to hear quite a bit from her when she was disappointed with me."

Not surprisingly, Deborah spent most of her younger years working as energetically as she could to earn praise from her parents. One consequence of this was that Deborah never really learned how to play. Self-indulgent recreation is an essential human skill that most of us learn when very young. My favorite example of this is one of my sons finger-painting at the age of three. He was not interested in the quality of the work or in how many pictures he could produce. He had no goal but his own joy. Deborah was too busy thinking about how to please others to spend much time on her own needs.

As an adult, Deborah continued to be hard working, reliable and detail-oriented. Her highest priority was the needs of those close to her and she occasionally skipped meals to get her many self-appointed tasks accomplished. "Sometimes I feel guilty if I go to sleep at night without having done everything on my list," she told me. Soon after her children were born, she was so busy she began to feel a constant painful tightness in her neck and shoulder muscles. After many years of this lifestyle, she conceded the possibility she needed a break, but she had never lived any other way.

Deborah's pain came from multiple stresses, though the most fundamental issue was her childhood experience. Getting approval from her mother always seemed just out of reach. Most children in her situation would go through a brick wall to satisfy their parent. Even that would likely be inadequate if the parent was Deborah's mother. Even worse, her mother's approval was doubly important because of the absence of Deborah's father and the indifference of her stepfather.

The lack of approval put Deborah on a treadmill she could not stop. Over a period of years, the stress led to depression. She was unaware that her increasing fatigue, difficulty sleeping and declining ability to cope were due to depression. She knew only that her stress level was getting worse and her frustration and exhaustion were increasing.

Deborah's treatment addressed all these issues. With counseling, she came to understand the connection between her childhood experience and her busy lifestyle. With that understanding, she found it much easier to modify her schedule. Deborah wrote a letter (that she never mailed) to her parents expressing her deepest thoughts and emotions. This helped her better comprehend the consequences of her early emotional neglect. She found five hours each week to develop her skills in self-indulgent relaxation. Eventually she became an avid bicyclist, even taking a week off to ride across the state of Oregon with a group of friends.

I gave her a Hero Award, explaining why the words were true. She taped the card to her bathroom mirror where she could see the words daily and kept it there for the next few years until she no longer needed it as a reminder.

We discussed medication for her depression symptoms, but she preferred to manage without that support. Her judgment proved to be correct as all her symptoms improved significantly over the next several months. Her primary physician then resumed her care, but sent a note two years later reporting that all her symptoms had gone away.

THE MOTHER-DAUGHTER BOND: BETTY AND CORINNE

Betty was just five years old on the day her mother did not come home from work. Betty's father noticed that a big suitcase and all of his wife's best clothes were gone. Betty never saw her mother again and for many years wondered what she had done to make her mother leave without warning. She became afraid to go to school and clung to her father as if he might leave too. It did not help when Betty's father told her she was acting like a baby.

Betty married when she was twenty and became just as dependent on her husband as she had been on her father. Her husband could count on hearing an emotional outpouring if he was late returning from his office or did not spell out his plans when he left the house. They had two children, Corinne and Cindy, but eventually Betty's husband grew tired of her endless needs. He moved to an apartment, filed for divorce and was soon living with a much younger girlfriend. Betty was devastated and turned to Corinne for emotional support. Corinne was four years old.

Corinne did her best to comfort her mother. She brought Betty things to cheer her, prepared food for her, took care of unpleasant chores around the house and was always alert to her mother's moods and needs. She did the same for her younger sister, Cindy, since Betty was usually unable to pay much attention to her children. Corinne's father did not show much interest in his children either, so whenever Corinne had a problem that needed the care of an adult she tended to rely on herself for a solution.

Betty's first suicide attempt occurred when Corinne was six. Corinne came home from playing with a neighbor and confronted the horrifying sight of her unconscious mother with a bloody neck wound. Corinne felt completely responsible and became determined never to let Betty harm herself again. From that day on, Corinne became extremely attentive to her mother's state of mind. Whenever Betty seemed unusually sad, Corinne would sleep with a pillow on the floor of her mother's bedroom "just to make sure she would be okay that night."

It was not enough. A few years later, Betty attempted suicide again, this time with pills. Several years after that she cut her throat and again, Corinne found her. Betty survived but after each of these traumas, Corinne redoubled her efforts to meet her mother's needs. When she slept in Betty's room, Corinne would wake up several times during the night and ask her mother how she was feeling.

When Corinne was in high school, Betty's doctors found medications that put an end to the suicide attempts though not to Corinne's worry. During this time Corinne also had to cope with Cindy, who was using drugs and was sexually active with multiple partners. Corinne lived at home while attending community college and continued living there after she got her first job as a ward secretary in a hospital. During these years she began having nightmares about finding her mother near death, had panic attacks at times, felt depressed, slept poorly, cried frequently, suffered from headaches and had frequent, painful abdominal cramps. The sight of a razor blade made her heart jump with fear. She went to the doctor about the headaches and cramps but no one asked about the many burdens in her life, her tests were normal and the treatments did not help much.

Corinne was still living at home at age thirty-two when she began dating Jeremy, a speech therapist who became her first real boyfriend. The following year he asked her to move into his house. Betty begged her daughter to stay at home "at least until you get married" and Corinne's headaches and abdominal pain became much worse. Somehow, though, with tears streaming down her face, she found a way to make the move.

Betty began telephoning Corinne two or three times a day, sometimes more on weekends. These calls were all about Betty's household needs, Betty's concerns about Cindy or Betty's emotional state. There was almost no discussion of Corinne's needs or feelings. Corinne listened patiently, tried to be helpful, declined to move back home and would always close by saying "I love you, Mom." Not surprisingly, Corinne's physical symptoms became progressively worse and when several more medical tests were normal, Corinne found herself in my office.

When we met, I could almost understand why none of her doctors had inquired about her personal life or her past. Although she seemed a little anxious and spoke quickly, she also smiled a lot, was not demanding that I find a solution to her symptoms and otherwise gave no reason to suspect the enormous pressure she had endured for thirty years.

Corinne's dysfunctional family life led to her suffering from post-traumatic stress, depression, panic attacks, and ongoing stress from the unrelenting demands of her mother, all of which combined to produce the physical symptoms. In addition, the constant attention Corinne gave to Betty and Cindy while she was growing up left Corinne unable to care for or even recognize her own needs. Consequently, she gave time and energy selflessly to Betty, to her job, to Jeremy and to her friends but only rarely to herself. The unrelieved stress led to her pains getting worse month by month.

After hearing her story, I explained the concept of stress illness but felt a little overwhelmed with the number and severity of her problems. I focused on Corinne's enduring childhood lesson that Betty needed constant attention or she would die. On three very traumatic occasions, Corinne felt she had failed Betty with nearly fatal consequences. Now Corinne was struggling to make a life for herself without neglecting Betty, who had always been her primary duty. In addition, the nightmares, crying, depression and panic attacks made Corinne feel emotionally inadequate.

However, despite enormous adversity, she had avoided the trap Cindy fell into of finding relief in drugs and promiscuous sex. Corinne had also educated herself, kept a steady job and formed a relationship with a man who held her hand throughout our interview and gave her solid support at home. Under the circumstances, this was almost miraculous and I told her so.

"You are like a champion body builder who has trained with heavy weights for years but is now asked to carry twice the usual load. Anyone would feel weak under those circumstances," I said.

Jeremy had a grade-school-age nephew named Trevor. I asked Corinne to imagine Trevor spending just one week in the same circumstances she had endured. "Imagine how difficult it would be watching Trevor try to cope, yet you lived in that environment for over thirty years," I said.

It was clear that Corinne would benefit from antidepressant medication and from mental health counseling and I arranged for both. However, the key would be for her to achieve a more reasonable level of separation from Betty and her endless demands. I advised Corinne that her symptoms were the body's way of telling her she needed a rest from Betty's phone calls. She began to hyperventilate at that idea but then remembered that Betty usually took care of Corinne when Corinne was ill. She concluded that because a physician was advising that Corinne needed rest, Betty would likely accept it.

I also gave Corinne a well-earned Hero Award, recommended that she keep a journal about her thoughts and emotions during the coming months and asked that she take five hours every week of personal time to learn how to enjoy and care for herself. With help from Jeremy, antidepressant medication and her counselor, Corinne made excellent progress. She accomplished the difficult task of forming a new self-image of a strong and thoughtful person to replace the old idea of herself as weak and ineffective. She discovered new interests and pleasures and understood she had earned the right to enjoy them.

These changes helped her develop firm boundaries in time and space between herself and Betty that she knew were essential to physical and mental health. As she accomplished these tasks, her physical symptoms diminished steadily and were nearly gone months later when Corinne accepted an engagement ring from Jeremy.

BELIEF SYSTEMS AND STRESS

Understanding a patient's religious beliefs is sometimes essential for successful treatment of stress illness. My religious opinions are not part of the discussion. The goal is to understand what my patients believe whenever this will help me care for them more successfully.

You are already familiar with the story of Carla, who feared God would deform her second baby as punishment for having her first pregnancy outside of marriage and for giving the first baby to an adopting family. Abandoned as a toddler by her mother, Carla was predisposed to a strong negative bias about herself and her relationship with God. This made it easy for Carla to believe in a God who would punish her. When I asked Carla to think about the act of giving up her first baby as similar to God giving Jesus to the world, she was able to include herself among those favored by God rather than among those selected for punishment.

You have also read about John, who believed in a powerful God. He prayed for his wife, Helen, to survive her severe liver disease and asked that he receive her itching in return for her life. Subconsciously John believed that as long as his own skin continued to itch, God would protect his beloved wife from a relapse. As with Carla, the emotional neglect John suffered as a boy made it easy for him to accept that he was more deserving of suffering than salvation. Bringing that point of view to light helped John to consider the idea that God saved Helen because of her own merits and because of John's prayer, but not because of John's continued suffering. This, combined with John's belief in a fundamentally loving God, was sufficient to relieve his itching.

The religious trigger of Barbara's illness is unique in the more than twenty years of my practice. She was thirty-four, worked for a company that made eyeglass lenses and for years had several symptoms that made no sense to the many doctors who tried to care for her. She told my nurse the doctors "aren't listening to me any more."

Barbara grew up on a farm near the Washington-Idaho border. Both her parents frequently used methamphetamines ("speed") and other drugs and fought bitterly. As the oldest daughter, Barbara managed the household and cared for her younger siblings whenever her parents could not. She remembered doing this work starting "when I was about six or seven." It was very natural for her to assume, even at that age, that she had an obligation to reduce the chaos in her home as much as she could. For a while, when life at home became too difficult, she could take her siblings to a neighboring farm. When the adult male in that household began fondling her, however, she felt trapped at home. These problems continued until Barbara graduated from high school with honors and moved to college on a scholarship.

Barbara suffered through a number of personal problems in her twenties and then, one day when she was thirty, "the Lord took me in his arms and saved me. I have never felt such love in my life." Soon after this heartfelt religious conversion, the stress illness symptoms began. This turned out to be an example of the Good Partner/Bad Illness syndrome, the partner being God. Barbara's new belief that she was worthy of God's love caused her to recognize more clearly how little she deserved to suffer as a child. She experienced strong, justifiable outrage about her suffering for the first time. On the other hand, her religious beliefs emphasized forgiveness. Almost as soon as she first felt the anger, she tried to suppress it by mentally pardoning her parents. The anger remained though, expressing itself through her physical symptoms.

I explained to Barbara that forgiveness can help some people move beyond their past (though for many others this is not essential). "But an honest pardon begins with a full accounting of all the transgressions," I told her. "I want you to make a list of all the problems you experienced as a child. Keep it with you as you think about whether you can truly forgive your parents for all the items on the list. I also think you should speak with a counselor at church or a therapist."

Barbara made the list and found a counselor to help her understand her feelings. She wrote about her experiences in a journal, met other people in her church who had overcome adversity in childhood and "prayed a lot." A few of her stress illness symptoms improved dramatically. Her other symptoms needed more time to make progress, but she could see they would be relieved in time.

One of my longest and most unusual interviews was with Michael. He was afflicted with frequent, violent coughing fits that defied years of attempts at diagnosis by allergists, lung specialists, throat specialists and gastroenterologists (who found he did not have stomach acid refluxing up his esophagus and spilling into his windpipe). Michael consumed large amounts of narcotic cough syrup every month but even that provided only partial relief.

Michael, forty-three and married for twenty years, worked as a produce buyer for a small food-processing firm founded and still directed by his father. As a child, he suffered significant verbal abuse from his father, who continued to criticize him at the office. Michael also had many symptoms of severe depression that were not improving despite medication and years of counseling by his psychiatrist.

Suddenly, in the middle of our interview and without any obvious connection to what we had been discussing, Michael made a statement about his worry that a "San Francisco element" might be coming to our area. I assumed his concern had to do with a shift to the left in Oregon politics and continued questioning Michael about sources of stress. Ten minutes later, he repeated the "San Francisco element" phrase, indicating it was something he thought was important. I asked him what he meant.

"Well, I mean, homosexuals," he replied.

"Are you concerned about homosexuals?" I asked.

"I am very much concerned," he replied.

"Why?"

"They're just a bad element. It says clearly in the Bible that sodomists should be cast out of society."

I had been asking him about stress in his life and now we were discussing the Biblical view of sodomy. Why had Michael directed our conversation to this subject?

"Do homosexuals contribute to your personal stress level?" I asked.

"Before I answer that question, I'm sorry, but I would feel more comfortable if I knew whether you were homosexual yourself," he replied. He had not asked this before telling me that gays were a "bad element," but now he wanted to know. This told me Michael was on the verge of sharing significant information. I let him know his question was not at all offensive, that I was not homosexual and that "I have been happily married to a wonderful woman since 1977."

"That's fine, thank you," he said, then coughed and cleared his throat several times. "When I was young I had some bad experiences," he went on.

I learned that between the ages of eight and ten he suffered several episodes of genital fondling by a small group of male teenagers in his neighborhood. There were no other episodes of sexual abuse in his life. These questions concluded my review of the stresses in his life, or so I thought. However, each time I tried to wrap up the interview and discuss my conclusions and plans for him, Michael brought up more details about stresses. His tone of voice became more agitated, but he added little of substance to what we had talked about already. The interview ran well beyond the appointment time, but Michael's manner was so intense I had a strong feeling I would learn something important if I listened to him for just a few more minutes.

Finally, he spoke the words I thought I might hear: "There is just one more thing." Michael rose from the chair, walked across the exam room, then returned to the chair and sat down. "When I was eighteen and nineteen, I had some more homosexual experiences."

"Were these unwanted as well?" I asked.

"No, they were voluntary on my part."

"How many times did this happen?"

"Oh, maybe seven or eight."

"Have you had any more since then?" I asked.

"No, none," he said firmly.

"I would like you to show me something, Michael. I am going to draw a line on a piece of paper and write the word 'male' at one end and 'female' at the other. I would like you to put a mark on the line showing me where your sexual preference lies. Is it toward the female end, toward the male end or somewhere in the middle of the line?"

I handed him my pen. I expected him to be in so much denial about his homosexuality that he would place the mark in the middle. He surprised me a little by placing the mark about 90 percent of the way toward the word "male."

"This must be an unbelievably difficult struggle for you," I responded, remembering his religious views and his marriage to a woman for twenty years. Michael coughed and cleared his throat several times, then nodded and said, "It isn't right for me to be this way." In the next several minutes, I learned that his wife Kristi was completely unaware of Michael's sexual preference. (Later I learned from Kristi that she and Michael had shared no significant sexual contact with each other during the last ten years.)

Even more difficult for Michael were his strong religious beliefs that condemned gays and lesbians and condoned removing them from society. He had already removed himself by living in a house deep in the Cascade Mountains. He often felt attracted to men he met, but had denied himself any physical or emotional relationship with another man since the age of nineteen. This powerful conflict had been torturing him for nearly twenty-five years.

Could these issues be the cause of Michael's violent fits of coughing? I was convinced this was the case, but relieving the cough was the only way to prove it. I believed his cough would persist indefinitely unless he achieved greater self-acceptance by reconciling his sexual preference with his religious views. Could either of these be changed? There are practitioners who claim to be able to change a patient's sexual preference, but they have little credibility with medical professionals. I looked for a way to help Michael within the framework of his religious beliefs. It seemed unlikely that his church would be a good resource since that group shared Michael's condemnation of sodomy. His psychiatrist, despite over five years of counseling Michael, was not aware he was gay so that did not seem to be a promising option either.

"I'm sure you have been trying for a long time to find a way to reconcile your sexual preference with your religious beliefs, Michael. Have you found any solutions?"

"I believe that you can love a man, and live with a man but not engage in sodomy," he replied. But never in the last twenty-five years had he come close to making that dream a reality. Michael also admitted to frequent strong temptation to have sexual contact with men and was bitter about his inability to overcome these desires.

I knew that a good outcome for Michael would be a long-term project and might never happen. Michael believed that God loved him, but also that God did not love his sexual preference. I concluded that his best option was to share the substance of our conversation with his psychiatrist. He agreed he would do that. His psychiatrist knew him well and I hoped their discussions might help Michael find a way for his religion and his sexual preference to co-exist peacefully. I saw Michael a few more times over the next five years, but his self-acceptance, his views on homosexuality and his cough did not change. Michael's depression grew deeper, he became a pathological gambler and he lost half a million dollars betting on sports. He went deeply into debt and then his father fired him from the company. One morning I saw his name in the newspaper. Hikers had found Michael's body at the bottom of a cliff, his death attributed to an accidental fall.

The emotional abuse Michael suffered from his father, the sexual abuse when he was nine, his severe depression and the irreconcilable conflict between his strong religious beliefs and his sexual preference for men combined to create wounds beyond our ability to heal. Years of counseling were unable to prevent his life from spiraling inexorably into tragedy.

Amanda was a petite twenty-four-year-old who possessed extraordinary mental toughness, but her body wailed in protest. For the last six months, pain across the middle of her chest was so intense that even the modest pressure of her bra was sometimes too much. Fortunately, the source of her illness was easy to find since a major stress occurred just before Amanda's symptoms began.

Amanda grew up within a religious community of about 250 people living in a twenty-square-mile area in the Midwest. One of the respected elders of this group molested Amanda about a half dozen times between the ages of ten and fourteen. Only his victims knew of his behavior and he remained a highly respected member of the church. When Amanda was twenty-three, she learned from a friend that the same man recently had molested two pre-teen sisters. Though she could tolerate her own suffering, Amanda became enraged that he was abusing others and undoubtedly had many victims about whom she knew nothing. She went to the church hierarchy with her story and was incredulous when they refused to believe her. She was told that her story was "impossible" and to pray for forgiveness for having falsely accused an honorable man.

Amanda then went to the police, which led to an investigation that stirred up outrage in everyone involved. Much to Amanda's dismay, the outrage focused on her and not the perpetrator.

"They excommunicated me from the church. My parents and my brothers disowned me. They would not speak to me. That was my whole world and they just closed the door," she said emotionally. This was when the chest pain began. She moved to south central Washington because she "heard it was nice" and tried to rebuild her life. Amanda practiced her religious beliefs alone.

I struggled to imagine what might help Amanda. She told the truth to men of faith whom she deeply respected and was soon cut off from every important person in her life. Fortunately, though she had lost trust in her church, her faith in the truth and in God remained strong. I knew a hospital chaplain not far from her home and he agreed to meet with her. They got along well and saw each other regularly. With his counseling, Amanda's chest pains improved steadily.

STRESS ILLNESS IN ADOLESCENTS: ROBERT

Robert was fifteen and over the past three weeks had experienced seven attacks of severe lower abdominal pain lasting several hours each. Robert's family was very concerned and he had already seen three doctors (without a diagnosis) before he came to my office. After a detailed discussion and review of his diagnostic tests, it seemed unlikely that his symptoms were due to an ulcer, inflammation or other visible abnormality.

When I asked if he had been under a lot of stress he slumped in his chair and a tear appeared in his eye as he said, "No, not really." Then the tear rolled down his cheek. "The other doctors asked me that, too, but there's really nothing," he added. More tears appeared.

I asked Robert to tell me a little about his life. He was a busy young man. His academic program was as rigorous as his school could provide and he was active in varsity sports, student government, the debate team and volunteer work. After all those commitments, he had little personal time. He was careful about his clothes and personal grooming and kept his room as well organized as the rest of his life. Robert described his parents as being supportive and affectionate, though he did add that his mother was "detail-oriented." Robert mentioned that even for something as simple as being late leaving the breakfast table for the school bus his mom might "go ballistic."

Both parents were interested in his grades and his other accomplishments at school. They clearly wanted the best for him, but as Robert went on talking it became clear that he was a slave to their expectations.

It was time for a key question. Had anything stressful occurred shortly before the onset of his abdominal pain? Robert recalled that he and his parents held a conference the night before his first pain attack. During this conference, it was "decided" that Robert was not staying on top of current events. His parents "recommended" he begin reading a weekly news magazine or business newspaper every day. Robert's schedule would not tolerate this last straw. He was caught between wanting to do what his parents felt was best and a personal schedule that was already at its limit. The abdominal pain was the result.

There was not time to conduct a full interview with the parents. My impression based on limited information was that they were successful in their careers because of hard work and attention to detail. It was no surprise they would apply these same values to raising their son. They paid close attention to every aspect of his life, wanted the best for him and taught him the rewards of hard work.

Ideally, a discussion with the parents would enable them to understand how these values can be taken too far when applied to children. A shift to less guidance and teaching and more cheering him on would provide the support Robert needed to find his own interests and values. He could then develop a better balance between work and play. Unfortunately, the appointment was too brief to bring the parents in from the waiting room and get to know them well.

Instead, we reviewed the many accomplishments that validated Robert's right to an opinion on how he spent his time. He agreed he was coping with much more than he realized. It was time to "just say no" to more stresses, to give himself more personal rest and relaxation and to feel justified in doing so.

An interesting discussion between Robert and his parents must have taken place because when I called a week later there had been no further attacks of pain. Six months later, I checked his record for medical appointments since our encounter and found only a routine visit to the optometrist.

Encouraging children to do their best is a key role for any parent. The fine line between appropriate supervision and inappropriate overburdening is never easy to find. When in doubt with a teen, a little more cheerleading and a little less guidance often will work out far better than many parents would guess.

STRESS ILLNESS IN ADOLESCENTS: JOAQUIN

Joaquin looked at me warily from the far side of a wide cultural gap. Now sixteen, he had spent most of his life in a tough Latino ghetto in California. At age ten he moved to Oregon with his mother and a few years later joined a gang. His school suspended him several times for threatening other students. He had an arrest record for petty larceny and defacing public property with graffiti.

Three months earlier, he began having attacks of severe abdominal pain. These would last anywhere from ten minutes to twelve hours. They often occurred during stressful events and stopped when the stress was over. For Joaquin, going to school was sometimes stressful enough to trigger an attack. When the school nurse sent him home, the pain was usually gone by the time he reached his front door.

Diagnostic testing by several pediatricians had been negative. Because of the close connection between his symptoms and stress, Joaquin received evaluations by three mental health therapists, yet his symptoms persisted. I knew I needed to learn much more about his life in order to help him.

Joaquin's parents divorced when he was three. His father was a violent, alcoholic drug abuser who regularly beat Joaquin's mother. He had knocked out some of her teeth, crushed bones in her hand, and put a gun to her head and in her mouth. He fathered a child with one of his nieces. Just before the divorce, Joaquin's father gave him alcohol to drink as a joke.

After the divorce, Joaquin saw his father on weekends for seven years until he moved to Oregon. He remembered his father telling him regularly "your mother is going to leave you just like she left me." He became fearful he might come home from school and find his mother had abandoned him, which was why he found going to school so stressful. After Joaquin moved to Oregon, his father never contacted him. Joaquin's father remarried, had more children and spent his time with his new family. Joaquin's anger at this rejection seethed. It did not take much for him to lose his temper and the school suspensions followed. One month before Joaquin's pain began, he decided to visit his father for the first time in six years. Anger dominated his emotions as he planned for the trip. He packed a baseball bat in his duffel bag with the idea he might want to beat his father with it.

As our discussion continued, I learned he had other motivations for the journey. He had heard that his father treated his new children well. In the back of his mind, Joaquin must have been wondering if his father was ready to treat him better. Was reconciliation possible?

When Joaquin arrived at his childhood home, he was bitterly disappointed. His father had not changed. He invited his son to drink alcohol and take drugs with him. There was no reconciliation and not much affection. At one point, he screamed at his father, "I will never love you."

The baseball bat stayed in the bag. Instead, he attacked his father's new car, driving it at top speed in second gear for several miles then suddenly shifting into reverse. Joaquin repeated this maneuver until he ruined the transmission.

Soon after returning to Oregon from this visit, Joaquin's abdominal pain began. He was certain he had no feelings for his father. "I don't care about him at all. He means nothing to me," he said angrily. I explained that we rarely feel for strangers the strong emotions he experienced during the visit with his father. Disappointment with those we care about generates the most powerful feelings.

Strong emotions that have no easy verbal outlet will find a way to make their presence known. Joaquin's emotions manifested themselves in his quick temper and the need to tell the world he existed through spray-painting his "tag" in public places. When he returned from the visit to his father, the anger level was even higher, unloading into his abdomen and causing severe pain.

I recommended he write about his father in a letter he would not mail. Joaquin said his writing skills were not strong, so we agreed he would speak into a voice recorder instead. He had also developed symptoms of depression: poor sleep, low energy and little appetite. I prescribed a relatively low dose of antidepressant medication. He returned to the mental health therapist with some new ideas to discuss. (The therapists he had seen earlier focused on his anti-social behavior and were not aware of the issues between Joaquin and his father.)

Joaquin had no further attacks of pain for a year, and then his antidepressant prescription ran out. A much milder version of the pain re-occurred until he contacted the office for a renewal of the prescription. After that, he remained well.

STRESS ILLNESS COINCIDING WITH A VISIBLE DISEASE

One of the most difficult diagnostic challenges a physician can face is when a disease with a visible cause and stress illness co-exist. This dilemma is particularly demanding when both conditions are causing the same symptoms. Success depends on evaluating and treating both problems simultaneously.

Toni was a large woman in her late twenties who nearly had unnecessary major surgery. Four years earlier, she developed ulcerative colitis, a condition in which the lining of the large intestine is raw with inflammation. Bloody diarrhea is the usual result when the disease flares up. Toni was fortunate that her colitis was mild and responded well to medication.

Two months before we met her colitis flared and a video exam of the lower bowel (colonoscopy) confirmed severe inflammation. Toni's doctor prescribed cortisone tablets to suppress the inflammation. This treatment is usually successful and after several weeks, the bleeding stopped. Unfortunately, her diarrhea was no better so her doctor put her in the hospital.

In the hospital, Toni received cortisone and nutrition by vein. She took nothing by mouth but broth, gelatin and water, allowing the bowel to rest. After ten days, her diarrhea was unchanged so her doctors scheduled an operation to remove the large intestine. Two days before the surgery Toni's doctor reviewed the case in detail one more time and discovered her diarrhea had an odd pattern. Toni might move her bowels six times in three hours and then not at all for eighteen hours. In someone with colitis who was eating very little this was unusual.

My colleague decided that Toni should have another video examination of the bowel and scheduled it for the next day. This time the colonoscopy showed that all the inflammation had healed! He canceled the surgery, cut the cortisone dose in half and asked me to talk to Toni about stresses in her life.

It turned out Toni was suffering through a major emotional crisis. As a girl, her father molested her repeatedly. Now, twenty years later, Toni recently had her first appointment with a therapist to discuss this issue and some problems in her marriage.

That first counseling session had not gone well. The therapist wanted to focus on the problems Toni was having in her life today. Toni wanted to talk about the past sexual abuse. She was very frustrated, cancelled the follow-up appointment with the therapist, felt she had nowhere to turn — and then the colitis flared up.

We spoke at length about the possibility that stress from long ago could be responsible for the diarrhea now that the colitis was under control. I assured her I would find a therapist who was experienced in helping clients recover from childhood abuse. I recommended she begin treatment for this problem by writing her thoughts and feelings in a journal.

Toni's diarrhea improved significantly after our discussion and she was able to leave the hospital the following day — the day originally scheduled for surgery. She followed up with a new counselor and made excellent progress.

All I had to do was mention the word stress to Randy and his story tumbled out.

"You might say I've been having a few problems at the office," he explained.

Randy was fifty-two with tangled, graying, blonde hair and a laugh that made me smile. He had worked for a large utility company for over twenty years. Like Toni, his ulcerative colitis appeared to be flaring up. Also like Toni, the pattern of his bowel movements was not typical for that disease: he felt fine two or three days each week and had frequent diarrhea on the other days.

Shortly before the symptoms began, a new employee joined the office and

Randy was her supervisor. The new employee, an attractive young woman, started working on a complex task with which she had little experience. Randy found himself spending more and more time training this woman and correcting her errors. After a few months, the new employee still had not mastered her job. Even worse, she did not seem too concerned about her repeated errors. Randy went to his supervisor and explained the situation. He expected the new employee to be fired or reassigned, but was shocked when his boss told him to continue training her.

Then word got out that Randy's supervisor and the incompetent but attractive new employee were having an affair that began before she was hired. Randy took the only option left: he went over the supervisor's head and demanded an investigation. In the bureaucratic company where Randy worked, this created a number of challenges and his diarrhea began soon afterward. The investigation was in full swing the day Randy sat in my office asking if he needed cortisone tablets.

Instead, we agreed to wait a few more weeks until the investigation finished. Fortunately, the new employee lost her job, the company demoted the supervisor and then reassigned him hundreds of miles away and Randy's diarrhea vanished.

CHAPTER 9

SEVEN KEYS TO TREATING STRESS ILLNESS

The most extreme conditions require the most extreme response, and for some individuals, the call to that response is vitality itself. The integrity and self-esteem gained from winning the battle against extremity are the richest treasures in my life.

– Diana Nyad, long distance swimmer

HELPING ONE OF MY PATIENTS TO OVERCOME STRESS ILLNESS IS A CHALLENGE FOR both of us. Helping a reader to accomplish this is even more difficult. To make the process a little clearer, I will present seven key ideas that, together, summarize the most important treatments. I suggest you re-read the keys from time to time as you move through different phases of leaving your symptoms behind.

Key 1 – Understand that your symptoms can be diagnosed and treated.

No matter how long you have been ill, the chances are excellent that you can find the cause of your symptoms and that useful treatment will be available. Begin with an evaluation by your doctor. Diseases other than stress illness can cause any symptom you have read about in this book. It is essential that you have a medical evaluation to investigate these other possibilities.

This leads directly to a question that troubles health care professionals as well as their patients: how many diagnostic tests are enough to be certain there is no other disease? When tests are repeatedly normal, the situation can be like trying to prove there are no fish in a lake. Will one more test reveal a diagnosis? Could a second opinion (or a third or fourth) put all the pieces together?

There are two answers to these questions. First, eventually we must rely on the clinician's judgment and experience to conclude that other diseases are unlikely. Second, it is entirely reasonable to consider stress as a possible cause of your symptoms even while the medical evaluation is in progress. If you identify and reduce sources of stress and find this helps your symptoms, and then learn that your diagnostic tests are normal, you and your physician can feel more confidence that stress is causing your illness.

Thousands of my patients have demonstrated the value of this approach. Once you understand this and believe you can feel better, you are ready for the next key.

Key 2 – Search for the sources of stress.

Most often, the stresses that cause symptoms are partly or completely hidden. You must become a detective and sift through evidence about your illness. Gather information including the date your symptoms began, how often they occur, their location in your body and any connections you can find to the people, places and events of your life. Write all this down under the heading "Illness Description."

The next step in your detective work is to create a "Stress Inventory." This is a list of every stress in your life from the past and present. Keep the list with you and add to it as new ideas come to mind. This is the first step in building an accurate understanding of everything you are coping with. When the list is complete, you might realize that the sheer number of items could explain your symptoms.

Next, use the illness description and the stress inventory to see if there is a close connection in timing between a particular stress and your symptoms. For example, Ellen (Chapter 1) always became ill in Mapleton while driving to visit her mother. You might also recall the woman whose symptoms came on after her mother, at the last minute, cancelled her promises to babysit. Another example is the patient who had stomach pain while driving to his difficult job but not while driving home. If you do find such a relationship, you will be well on your way to understanding the cause of your illness.

Most of the time, however, there is no direct connection in timing between a stress and the symptoms. In the majority of cases, illness results from an accumulation of the many stresses in your inventory or from a long-term emotional process. Sometimes the stress is obvious, such as a spouse or partner who hits or slaps you or controls your life. In other people, the stresses are more difficult to find. This is particularly true for childhood stress where a significant lowering of the child's self-esteem persists into the adult years. Explore this possibility by considering whether your childhood resembled any of the families described in earlier chapters. Ask yourself if it would be disturbing to watch a child grow up in the same way you did. If so, then you have found an important source of stress.

Finally, look again at the chapters describing the characteristic symptoms of depression, post-traumatic stress and anxiety to see if any apply to you. Films and television can mislead the public by portraying these conditions in dramatic ways. We see a depressed person threatening to jump from a high ledge. A combat veteran with post-traumatic stress flinches when a balloon bursts nearby. An anxious person draws the attention of a crowd by panicking and then breathing into a paper bag. Any of these problems can happen to people with these conditions but most of the time the symptoms are not so obvious. Many patients suffer quietly for years, unaware that beneficial treatment is readily available. If you are uncertain, ask your doctor or a mental health professional.

Key 3 – Care for yourself.

Symptoms can be the body's way of asking you to care for yourself. Begin your response to this message from your body by looking at your inventory of stresses. Try to find two or three items on the list that you can improve. If you succeed, those changes in your life might be enough to reduce some of your symptoms. This will encourage you to make even more changes.

Next, recognize when stress is a by-product of too many demands or being stretched too thin. Commit to specific steps for creating boundaries so you will have time for yourself. Tell your loved ones that you will be taking five hours per week for personal self-care. Tell them you will need their support to manage tasks you might otherwise be doing. (When trying to focus on yourself, the last thing you need is worry about work piling up at home, but I know that some of my patients are unable to avoid this completely.) Use this time to find activities that are so enjoyable you cannot wait to do them again next week.

Do not worry if you have no idea how to use personal time. My patients who need this time the most usually have no idea what to do at first. Give yourself permission to take a few months of trial and error to find the experiences that work best for you. Be assured that everything you try will teach you more about your needs. The process is similar to learning to ride a bicycle. You won't get it right early on but persistence leads to success.

Be prepared to feel guilty when you take personal time. Accept that you deserve to care for yourself as much as you care for others. Recognize that you are merely adding your name to the list of people for whom you provide care. Remember that you cannot be useful to others if you work until you become ill. Understand that even if you did not have enough opportunities to learn self-care as a child, you can acquire this essential skill at any age.

Another approach to the guilt, if you experienced hardship in the past, is to give yourself a Hero Award (see Chapter 3) to recognize the quality of character needed to overcome adversity. Place the award where it can be seen daily and keep it there until you no longer need the reminder. This will help you think about yourself in a positive way, which will make it easier to find guilt-free time to care for yourself.

This key seems so simple. However, for my patients who need it most, it can be quite challenging. If you are one of these patients, be encouraged by two ideas. First, this key is such a powerful healer that even patients hospitalized for severe symptoms eventually have had complete relief from using it. Second, in many patients this key is the only treatment needed to relieve their stress illness.

Key 4 – Get right by writing.

Remember that physical symptoms often result when the brain unloads trapped emotions into the body. Converting those suppressed feelings into words – spoken into a recorder or written on paper – provides the brain with a different outlet. Writing, in particular, has a way of revealing emotions people did not suspect they had. For many patients, the more they can express in words, the less the brain will need to release into the body.

I have already recommended the stress inventory, a writing exercise that starts the healing process for most patients. Childhood stress survivors should be sure to include their early difficult experiences in the inventory. This will begin the process of linking emotions from childhood to verbal coping skills.

Most people with stress illness, when they feel ready, also can benefit from writing in a journal (or talking into a recorder) about difficult experiences and people in their lives. Expression of thoughts and emotions should be as honest and complete as possible. The amount and frequency of writing (or speaking) is less important. Patients should trust themselves in this area because when they *feel* ready to do this, they usually *are* ready.

Another useful exercise, if you are a childhood stress survivor, is to write a letter to people whom you cared about but who also caused significant problems for you as a child. This could be a parent who lived with you or one who was absent for much of your life. It could also be a stepparent, an older sibling or a relative. My patients rarely mail the letters and usually keep them in a safe place but sometimes they burn them. One of my patients put the letter to her father into a toy boat and pushed it into the ocean near the place where he had drowned. Another patient took the letter to her parent's grave and read it aloud. Another idea is to imagine yourself observing a child who is enduring the same difficulties you experienced. Write (or speak) to that child to express your feelings and provide advice on how to cope. You might also imagine your parents magically transformed into loving and supportive people and write (or speak) about how that might have changed your early life and changed you.

All of these ideas will help reveal hidden emotions, which is the first step toward understanding them. Once this process starts, it strengthens over time and gradually reduces the need for the mind to unload emotional stress into the body. Physical symptoms will improve as a result.

Key 5 – Use appropriate therapies.

Mental health treatment is an important resource for many stress illness patients. Among these are childhood stress survivors and people with certain forms of current stress such as marital or sexual problems. There is also good research showing the value of medications or counseling (or both) for most patients suffering from depression, post-traumatic stress or an anxiety disorder. If symptoms from these conditions are interfering with your life, if you have any thoughts of harming yourself, if you have an addiction or an eating disorder or are experiencing hallucinations, then let your doctor or a mental health practitioner know right away.

A decision about using medication should occur after an evaluation by a qualified professional and a discussion of benefits and side effects. For many patients, successful treatment can result from counseling alone. A trial of counseling also can be offered to patients who would likely benefit from medication, but who are reluctant to take something that affects brain function.

If a doctor recommends medication for you, it can be reassuring to know that the benefits derive from correcting abnormal levels of essential chemicals (neurotransmitters, Chapter 6) in the nervous system. This is a little bit like giving insulin to a diabetic. The goal is to restore chemical balance to enable the system to function as nature intended. In some patients, it can be difficult or impossible to overcome depression, post-traumatic stress or an anxiety disorder unless the brain's chemical balance is improved.

In choosing a mental health practitioner, be sure to ask about their experience treating problems similar to your own. In particular, childhood stress survivors benefit from counseling by those who have an interest in this problem and therefore have special experience helping overcome poor self-esteem, unexpressed anger, lack of self-care skills and many other issues common in these patients. For some people with strong religious beliefs, pastoral counseling and spiritual support will suffice either by itself or in combination with mental health treatment.

Key 6 – Overcome hidden resistance.

Many stress illness patients have issues they do not fully comprehend that can undermine their best efforts to get better. Finding and removing these hidden impediments will significantly enhance the effectiveness of other treatments. Mental health counseling often plays an important role in this process.

First, it is essential to recognize false beliefs about yourself. Most of these have their origins in adverse childhood experience. In dysfunctional homes, children frequently feel incompetent, unworthy of affection, not in control of who touches their body, powerless to change their environment, unable to change themselves and obligated to meet the needs of others before attending to needs of their own. People subjected to these feelings in childhood often carry them into their adult years. If this happened to you, recognize that you can rid yourself of these false concepts. Start by understanding that these beliefs have nothing to do with the person you are meant to be and everything to do with your early environment. The self-care and writing keys will help with this work. You should also respect the heroic personal qualities that enabled you to survive. If you have any doubt that it took heroism to survive, imagine that a child you care about is struggling with the same family environment. It is not easy to change assumptions that took root at an early age. However, my patients have found that overcoming false beliefs is not as difficult as surviving the home that planted those ideas in the first place.

A second hidden obstacle to change is parents who are unable to respect your accomplishments. Though difficult, try to understand that this reflects only their shortcomings, not yours. This can take time if you have spent your life trying to live up to their expectations. It can help to imagine yourself imposing the same criticism and impossible expectations on a child you know. When you imagine the hurt expression in that child's face, it will give you a clearer understanding of what you have endured.

Third, if you are in a relationship where the affection, support and respect are strong, mutual and balanced but you feel unworthy of it, look back at the achievements of your life. Then consider whether your partner simply sees you as you are, not as others have made you feel in the past. This work, too, benefits from the self-care and writing keys.

Fourth, if you are in a relationship where the affection, support and respect are not mutual and balanced, then review the achievements of your life and consider whether you deserve better. Many of my patients are in relationships where they receive much less than they give. They tend to accept this because of negative self-concepts they have carried since they were children. Replacing these beliefs with more accurate ideas about self worth will either help the relationship change for the better or make it clear that the relationship should end.

Identifying and coping with these hidden barriers to growth is essential to overcoming stress illness. This is not easy so do not assume you are a failure if you cannot eliminate these problems right away. This is not a reflection on you but is, instead, an indication of the severity of stress you are coping with.

Key 7 – Become the person you were always meant to be.

This is the ultimate goal. The first six keys will lead you here by relieving symptoms and by improving self-understanding, which is essential for growth. This is why many patients find that the changes they make to relieve stress illness also free them to achieve their potential. They become aware of how certain people or experiences pushed them down stressful pathways and this awareness supports making new choices.

For example, my patients from a dysfunctional childhood begin their healing by recognizing that their early environment led to false self-concepts. When they are free from these untrue assumptions, they can look at themselves with greater accuracy, sympathy and understanding. With this foundation, they are less accepting of disrespectful treatment, more willing to care for themselves, more likely to become involved in mutually supportive relationships and better prepared to develop and pursue their dreams.

The stress inventory is another technique that enhances self-knowledge by clarifying a patient's full range of problems. Many people have an incomplete understanding of this because they have always considered the issues individually, never collectively. Reducing even a few of the sources of stress provides more freedom for personal growth.

Two other aids to learning about yourself are setting aside regular personal time and mental health treatment. Time spent in self-care can provide opportunities for growth that you probably would not encounter otherwise and counseling can have a positive influence on your goals and beliefs. If medication is prescribed, this can help correct neurotransmitter imbalance that is limiting healthy mental functioning.

All these resources build on the strengths that enabled you to overcome stress in the past. They help remove distortions caused by adverse people and events. With their support, you can grow to become the person you were always meant to be.

I will conclude with a true story that, in its own way, summarizes the process of relieving stress illness. Six or seven centuries ago in Ayuthaya, the great capital of Siam, skilled artisans used over five tons of gold to cast a ten-foot-high statue of the Buddha. In the 1700s, to conceal its value from Burmese invaders, temple workers covered it with a thin layer of plaster. However, the need for the disguise outlived those who knew the secret and the full beauty of the statue remained hidden for the next two hundred years. In the 1950s, damage to the plaster occurred during transport from a warehouse to the humble Wat Traimit temple in Bangkok. A worker noticed a gleam where the damage had occurred and now the Golden Buddha inspires awe and reverence in everyone who sees it. My own encounter with the statue sometimes comes to mind as I try to help stress illness patients remove the plaster so they can see the gold.

PART III
CONNECTIONS

We are to regard the mind not as a piece of iron to be
laid upon the anvil and hammered into any shape,
nor as a block of marble in which we are to find
the statue by removing the rubbish, nor as a receptacle
into which knowledge may be poured; but as a flame
that is to be fed, as an active being that must be
strengthened to think and to feel, to dare and to do.

– Mark Hopkins

CHAPTER 10

STRESS ILLNESS
IN LOVED ONES

*The Family — that dear octopus from whose tentacles
we never quite escape nor, in our inmost hearts, ever
quite wish to.*

– Dodie Smith

STRESS ILLNESS CAN BE ALMOST AS FRUSTRATING FOR FAMILY MEMBERS AS IT IS FOR the patient. When a medical evaluation by a physician fails to identify a cause for symptoms and one or more of the five types of stress is present, treatment directed at the stress can take time to produce results. During this period, the right kind of support from loved ones not only makes life easier, but also helps the patient recover more quickly.

The "right kind of support" will differ depending on the nature of the stress. Individuals suffering from present day stresses clearly will benefit from anything that relieves their most pressing concerns. For example, many of my patients suffering from lack of personal time have been fortunate to have a spouse who took on enough tasks or roles to enable their loved one to have personal time every week. Many went even further and insisted that their loved one not use their personal time for anything but self-care. Since old habits do not change easily this requires a lot of patience, but steadfast adherence to the message will eventually lead to lasting positive changes.

Depression, anxiety and post-traumatic stress are associated with changes in brain wiring and chemistry and take time to improve. Moral support, encouragement and relief of present day stresses (as much as possible) while the patient is undergoing treatment are always helpful.

Recovery from childhood stress also responds to support from a loved one. The loss of self-esteem experienced as a child has no better antidote than love, respect and kind words. Helping abuse survivors understand that what they learned about themselves as children was false is the key to leaving the past behind.

In other situations, the best way to support a loved one is not so clear. For example, some individuals refuse to follow a recommendation for mental health counseling. Part of the issue is the stigma associated with mental health treatment. I remind my patients that mental health practitioners are specialists in brain chemistry and wiring and that, at times, I need to refer to them as I would to any other specialist. If the symptoms resulted from a chemical imbalance in the heart and I referred them to a heart specialist, there would be no hesitation about keeping the appointment. There should be no difference with a mental health clinician because the brain is a flesh and blood organ like any other.

This might not be the only concern about seeing a mental health specialist. For example, there could be fear of divulging deeply personal and troubling information. When I hear "I don't want to discuss that right now," I have to respect my patient's wish. Encouraging patients with this concern to write in a private journal can help initiate communication about even the most difficult problems.

Some child abuse survivors are reluctant to accept help from a mental health clinician for another reason. A person who is struggling to regain self-esteem demolished in childhood might view acceptance of psychological therapy as evidence of inability to solve personal problems. For these people, going to a therapist might feel like admitting personal inadequacy. Is it possible to overcome this resistance? In the box are some ideas that can help a stress illness patient see mental health counseling more favorably.

Ideas About the Value of Mental Health Counseling

- Stress sufficient to produce physical symptoms is a great burden. It need not be carried alone. If you needed to maneuver a canoe across a lake with the wind blowing hard in your face, you could do it alone but it would be easier if you had some help.

- If you had a heart problem, wouldn't you take charge of the situation by seeing a heart specialist?

- Would it have helped you as a child, if a parent who created problems had sought help from a counselor? If you had been in the doctor's office when the doctor recommended a mental health appointment for your parent, would you have recommended that they go? What would you have said if your parent declined or went for just one visit?

- Imagine that your best friend's spouse comes to you expressing concern about your best friend. The spouse tells you your best friend is having problems that are causing emotional pain for the family. The problems turn out to be all the same things you are hearing about yourself from your spouse, friends, co-workers or doctor. The spouse tells you a doctor recommended mental health treatment for your best friend. You agree to talk to your best friend. What will you say?

- If a stranger, neighbor or relative caused emotional pain in your family, would you take action to put a stop to it? If it happens to be you who is causing pain for your loved ones, who better to put a stop to it?

Remember that a good message, presented in a loving and supportive but patient and persistent way, might not produce any sign of change until the moment a person decides to act in agreement with the message.

A few spouses and partners of stress illness patients face verbal or physical violence. (This occurs less often than you might expect because it is the nature of stress illness that anger is internalized and not externalized.) If there is violence in the relationship then the safety of everyone living in the household takes precedence over other concerns. Review the situation with a social worker as soon as possible to become familiar with local support options.

When the stress illness patient is an adolescent and you are the parent then you should consider the uncomfortable possibility that you might be contributing to the illness. This can be obvious when the household has a parent, stepparent, guardian or other adult authority figure that commits abuse, is violent or abuses alcohol or drugs.

For many of my teen patients, though, the source of stress is not so easy to detect. The parents of these afflicted adolescents want only the best for their child. They know the world can be a tough place, they want to prepare their child every way they can and they regularly suggest ways for their child to improve. Even for teens without serious personal problems, the number of opportunities for helpful advice is nearly endless:

- Personal hygiene
- Weight (too fat or thin)
- Table manners
- Bedroom cleanliness
- Clothing choices
- Study habits
- Sleeping habits
- Grades
- Academic testing scores
- Time spent with personal electronics or television
- Musical instrument or athletic practice time
- Shortcomings in artistic performance or on the athletic field
- Choice of friends
- Automobile driving technique
- Spending habits
- Music preferences
- College or career plans

Many parents of adolescents with stress illness never cease finding room for improvement in these areas. It is all too easy for well-meaning parents to create an atmosphere of unrelenting pressure. It would be an interesting experience for these parents to have the tables turned and have an authority figure follow them through their day and comment (supportively and with the best intentions) every time a shortcoming was observed. For most parents it would not be long before they were ready to boot the authority figure out their front door. For another example, imagine you are at home after a tough day. Would you rather that a loved one listen sympathetically and supportively and offer you a favorite beverage or would you prefer instruction intended to improve your time management skills?

Most teenagers work very hard to please their parents, even if it ties their guts in a knot. Parents also tend to forget that teens, while outside the home environment, regularly confront real or imagined personal shortcomings in such areas as:

- Physical attractiveness
- Athletic prowess
- Sexual experience
- Artistic talent
- Popularity
- Academic ability
- Financial resources
- Clothing
- Personal transportation

The pressure can build without anyone recognizing it and with nothing but the best intentions on the part of everyone involved. This is particularly true for parents who grew up in a dysfunctional home, where close attention to detail can be essential for survival. Often they become parents who focus especially carefully on the details of their children's lives.

To lessen these problems while maintaining an environment in which your child can excel, it might help to examine what motivates you toward excellence. Recall that the more you enjoy doing something, the more likely you are to spend time at it. If you love running and teamwork, you are more likely to play soccer or football than shoot pool. If you love numbers but have only average hand-eye co-ordination, then you are more likely to work in finance than heart surgery. Even more important, when someone praises your efforts, the activity becomes even more enjoyable and your motivation to continue and to improve is increased.

Teens feel the same way. They are trying to find and understand their talents and are searching for the best fit between their abilities and what the world offers. Hearing they have done well motivates them, learning they could have done better does not. As a parent, find every opportunity to share sincere positive comments for your adolescent's accomplishment or improvement. A word or two is often enough. Try to achieve the highest possible ratio of praising to advising. Certainly you should know what your child is doing and set limits that ensure safety (and a reasonable amount of sleep), but beyond that try to minimize how often you question or restrict them. This shows your trust in the teen's judgment and builds their self-confidence. Then when the world throws something new at them, confidence and self-esteem will be their foundation for adapting to and overcoming the challenge.

Every teen will have opportunities to engage in irresponsible, illegal or dangerous behavior when you are not there to supervise. They will be more likely to walk away from these situations if they have the self-confidence to resist peer pressure and care enough about how you would feel. They will care about you if they see that you:

- Set reasonable limits
- Know about your children's choices but let them make decisions as often as is consistent with safety and family needs
- Are their cheerleader more often than their supervisor
- Let them know that making mistakes is part of life, has been part of your life, and is not a negative reflection on character

With these ideas in mind, the adolescent will perceive your trust and support. The resulting affection for you and confidence in himself or herself will translate into better personal choices, better preparation for life and relief from a major source of stress.

CHAPTER 11
STRESS ILLNESS AND THE HEALTH CARE SYSTEM

The work of medicine, in considerable part, rests on the doctor's ability to listen to the stories that patients tell, to make sense of those often chaotic narratives of illness, to inspect and evaluate the listener's response to the story told, to understand what these narratives mean, and to be moved by them.

– Rita Charon

MILLIONS OF PEOPLE HAVE STRESS ILLNESS AND MOST OF THEM DO NOT RECEIVE the same quality of care as patients with cancer, hepatitis, hardening of the arteries or other diseases. This section, written primarily for health care professionals (clinicians, educators and administrators) but also for the general reader, will review changes in care delivery that could improve management of stress illness.

Why is the level of care for stress illness so poor? The problem begins with a lack of training. Doctors spend years learning about the visible abnormalities that will explain their patients' symptoms. These abnormalities can be plainly visible like a rash, hidden like a brain tumor, microscopic as in infection or biochemical as in sickle cell anemia but they can all be seen with the right instrument or test. Unfortunately, most medical students spend far less time learning to manage symptoms with the invisible cause of stress.

I wish it were possible to invent a blood test for stress illness. If such a test came into existence, medical schools would immediately devote as much class time to stress illness as is now devoted to diseases of the lungs, heart, kidneys or liver. (Although when you think about it, the absence of a diagnostic test is an even better reason for medical schools to spend time teaching about stress illness since the lack of a test makes it more difficult to diagnose.)

Another reason for the poor care of stress illness is the amount of time needed for diagnosis. With illness caused by visible abnormalities, the doctor needs to answer the question: "What is the disease?" This can be time-consuming enough in many cases. In stress illness, the key question can be "What difficult experiences have you had and how did they affect your life?" This can take much longer to answer and in many medical practices, the extra time needed to gather this information might not seem available. Of course, time spent answering this question will usually lead more rapidly to the correct diagnosis and thereby save time in the end.

Another issue is that assessment of visible illness and stress illness involve two different styles of thinking. Many doctors working in diagnostic medicine think primarily in physiological terms. This is analogous to an engineer's approach to the body. Diagnosis and treatment of stress illness, however, often require psychological thinking. Outside of the mental health profession, few doctors have had much training in psychological assessment and most clinicians are not comfortable doing it.

For all these reasons, correcting deficiencies in the care of stress illness must begin with the training of doctors. A key skill is empathy, which is often confused with sympathy or compassion. Empathy means using imagination and experience to feel personally the patient's emotional perspective. "How must this patient feel?" is a question that usually needs an answer for successful diagnosis and treatment of stress illness.

The story of John and his unusual itching (Chapter 2) is a good example. To understand his illness meant recognizing what it must be like for a man of strong religious faith to grow up emotionally neglected, to find the love of his life in Helen and then almost to lose her to illness twice. When he told his story, it came across as a seemingly random series of events and emotions that mixed the past with the present. Most patient histories are similar. Empathy was essential to organizing the pieces of his medical history in a way that led to understanding his stress.

Learning empathy takes time and practice. Those who teach medicine should model clinical empathy for their students. Another useful learning method is to write about an illness from the perspective of the afflicted patient, preferably just after the encounter. Achieving empathy with one patient will make connecting with the next patient that much easier.

A second key skill is interview technique. In teaching doctors about interviewing, I emphasize beginning with open-ended questions and interrupting the patient as little as possible. During the interview, doctors should acquire a full description of:

- When the symptoms began
- The frequency of the symptoms
- Patterns in the timing of the symptoms with respect to hour of the day, day of the week, time of year and relationship to personal activities and interactions with others. This information is the foundation for later being able to find associations between events in an individual's life and the activity of their symptoms. One of my patients, for example, developed intestinal symptoms in 1980, in 1991 and in 1998. She had none of these symptoms at any other time in her life. Later in our discussion, I learned that in 1980 she moved two thousand miles from her childhood home to take her first job. Her bowel problems re-occurred in 1991 during a divorce. The symptoms relapsed again during her second divorce in 1998. These were by far the most stressful events in her life. Knowing the timing of her symptoms was essential to seeing the connection.

The next step is to make it clear to the patient that symptoms caused by stress result from a physiological process no different in principle from processes that produce ulcers or tumors. Once this concept is accepted, people are much more willing to discuss sources of stress. The earlier in the diagnostic process this discussion happens, the more willing the patient will be to participate and the sooner the correct diagnosis will occur.

After gaining the cooperation of the patient, the doctor should inquire about stress the patient is experiencing now or recently. This could include personal issues, problems in the family or workplace and insufficient personal time. With a clear idea of the timing of their symptoms, it is often possible to connect these stresses to the symptoms.

For example, one of my patients reported stomach problems mostly in the mornings. It turned out to be primarily weekday mornings. Then it turned out to be weekday mornings while in the car driving to work. Then he related how stressful his job had become. Finally, he recognized he had no stomach problems while driving home from work.

Next, doctors should inquire about any traumatic events that occurred in the past. By keeping in mind the timing of the symptoms, the doctor might find a relationship between the trauma and the onset of the symptoms. (The symptoms could have begun on an anniversary of the traumatic event, for example.)

One patient of mine recalled the exact day that his chest pain began. It turned out to be the fifth anniversary of his father's murder, which was still unsolved. He had never made the connection until I asked about traumatic events, learned about his father's violent death and learned the date he died.

Another patient mentioned during discussion of her symptoms that she often awoke at precisely 1:08 AM. This happened a few nights each week for several years. A few months before her illness began her husband and parents were in a motor vehicle that crashed, killing her mother and husband. Her father recovered after weeks in intensive care. The car had crashed at 4:08 AM, but three time zones to our east in Connecticut. She was waking up at the precise moment of the accident and her illness was due to post-traumatic stress.

Next should be a review of the symptoms of depression. This can be a subtle illness. Many who have this condition do not feel depressed. If a patient has many of the symptoms of depression but does not feel depressed, then I speak in terms of a chemical imbalance in the nervous system being responsible for their symptoms. I often make an analogy with diabetes, which is also due to a chemical imbalance. This makes the whole concept more comprehensible and eases acceptance of treatment. Trying to convince a patient they have depression when they do not feel depressed is usually unnecessary and counter-productive.

Sometimes a patient's most prominent symptom of depression is being unable to cope as well with their usual stresses. You might recall a patient discussed earlier who had lived in a windy area known as the Columbia River Gorge for fifteen years. In the past year, he had become intolerant of the sound of the wind blowing around his home. That was, in fact, the problem that he wanted solved. His exact words: "I just can't take the wind anymore, Doc." For fourteen of the fifteen years there had been no such problem. With antidepressant medication, his concern went away completely.

Doctors should also ask about symptoms of anxiety, including symptom episodes associated with fear. Asking about difficulty breathing or numbness and tingling in the limbs that might signify hyperventilation is also important. If the doctor suspects an anxiety disorder, they should ask how the patient feels when they are frightened and see if those feelings match any of the symptoms.

More than half of my patients with stress illness grew up in dysfunctional families. Doctors should learn as much about childhood stresses as the patient feels comfortable sharing. It is important to remember that some survivors of dysfunctional homes learned not to express their emotions or not to feel the emotions at all. Consequently, they might not fully comprehend the impact of the negative aspects of their early years. Many of my patients, for example, initially denied that their childhood experience was difficult.

Repeated lowering of the child's self-esteem is the common denominator for childhood stress that can lead to illness in adults. The interview should search for events in the patient's early years that might have had this effect. Verbal, physical, sexual or emotional abuses are the most common. Parental drug abuse, domestic violence, excessively high parental standards or bullying by peers are also common in the childhood histories of adults with stress illness.

It is also useful to look for certain personality traits that are frequent in adult survivors of a dysfunctional childhood home. These are evidence of a long-term impact of the early environment. For example, does the patient provide evidence that he or she is a perfectionist or self-sacrificing? Is there a history of long-term relationships with partners who treated the patient badly? Is self-esteem still low? Is there a history of addiction, eating disorders, mental health problems, self-mutilation, anger outbursts or promiscuity? The more of these the doctor finds, the more likely it is that the childhood environment was damaging enough to produce stress illness.

Also in childhood stress survivors, look for a positive event that occurred near the time symptoms began. It is quite common for stress illness symptoms to occur soon after such an event (recall the "Good Partner/Bad Illness" syndrome). The positive event is not necessarily a new and better personal relationship. One patient developed symptoms after receiving the "Person of the Year" award at his company. Another became ill when she received her Ph.D. degree after many years of personal sacrifice. These life-affirming events create turmoil by their stark contrast with prior negative treatment and low self-esteem.

In summary, while the medical diagnostic process tries to "find the disease," the process used in diagnosing stress illness tries to understand the patient as a person. An excellent way to gain this understanding is to ask about the five types of stress. Doctors will gain confidence diagnosing stress illness as they become more experienced asking these questions.

When stress illness is a potential cause for a patient's symptoms, it is appropriate for the doctor to recommend one or more of the treatment measures described in this book. Tailoring these recommendations to the particular stresses affecting each patient is best. If the symptoms respond positively to these techniques, then confidence in the diagnosis is justifiably increased.

Training doctors to better recognize the presence of stress illness is part of the answer to helping the millions of people with this disease. Because so much of stress illness is psychological in nature, another essential step in managing this population is integration of mental health professionals into primary care medical practice. In modern medicine, we have specialists for every organ system but no one who specializes in stress illness in spite of the vast numbers who are afflicted. Having a trained mental health counselor immediately available for consultations, assessment and treatment of patients with stress illness would make an enormous difference. (In my medical group, the usual qualification for these practitioners is a master's degree in a mental health field.) Combining the counselor's psychological expertise with the medical knowledge of the primary care clinician — often during the same office visit – enables investigation of the full range of causes of symptoms. Even better, patients perceive this as an extension of their primary medical care instead of a diversion to mental health.

Integrating a mental health clinician into primary care (I call them stress medicine specialists) also allows for regular interaction with the medical clinicians. Each type of provider becomes more skilled in the other's area of expertise. Correct diagnosis and appropriate treatment is easier and faster and the huge blind spot between the medical and the psychological in patient care begins to close. My medical group and several others have begun this practice in the last few years and it has proven highly useful and popular with doctors and patients. Most primary care practices with at least three or four clinicians could offer great benefit to their patients by adding a mental health professional.

Health education also plays a vital role in the management of stress illness. Providing patients with an understanding of their condition enables many to care for themselves. The task for a health care system then becomes one of delivering this information to those who need it. Options for delivering additional information include:

- A brochure introducing the stress illness concept (suggested title: *Is Stress Making You Ill?*) to place in exam rooms.
- A Behavioral Health Questionnaire that screens for a variety of forms of stress coupled with information similar to that in the brochure.
- A group lecture/discussion to introduce the concepts in this book (suggested title: *Stress Medicine Group Appointment*). This has been very popular with patients. The appendix lists the medical journal reference for my article about this lecture.
- A web site such as my own www.stressillness.com.
- A short video program (suggested title: *Is Stress Causing Your Illness?*)
- "Life Skills Classes" to cover such subjects as stress management, depression, low self-esteem and adult children of dysfunctional families.

Resources like these have enabled thousands of patients with stress illness to learn how to cope and many patients have completely recovered from their illness. I look forward to the day when management of stress illness will be just as routine and successful as that of any other medical condition.

APPENDIX
PUBLICATIONS

THIS BOOK HAS INTRODUCED YOU TO THE FIVE TYPES OF STRESS AND THEIR connections to physical symptoms. Many of my readers will benefit from learning more about the specific stresses they are coping with. Here is a list of excellent references to get you started.

Childhood Stress

Adult Children of Alcoholics: Expanded Edition by Janet Woititz

Betrayal of Innocence: Incest and Its Devastation by Susan Forward and Craig Buck

Opening Up: The Healing Power of Expressing Emotions by James Pennebaker. About therapeutic writing. Also helpful for trauma survivors.

A Private Family Matter by Victor Rivers. Moving personal story of recovery from child abuse.

Current Stress

The Betrayal Bond by Patrick Carnes. How to recognize exploitive relationships and then remove yourself from them.

The Healthy Mind, Healthy Body Handbook by Sobel and Ornstein

The Relaxation & Stress Reduction Workbook by M. Davis et al

Depression

The Depression Workbook: A Guide for Living with Depression and Manic Depression, Second Edition by Copeland and McKay

Ten Days to Self-Esteem by David Burns

Anxiety Disorders

The Anxiety & Phobia Workbook by Edmund Bourne

Post-Traumatic Stress

I Can't Get over It: A Handbook for Trauma Survivors by Aphrodite Matsakis

For Health Care Professionals

Caring for Patients by Alan Barbour

Mind, Body and Medicine by Raphael Melmed

From Detached Concern to Empathy: Humanizing Medical Practice by Jodi Halpern

Clarke DD. "Functional Gastrointestinal Symptoms: A New Approach Using a Stress Illness Diagnosis Clinic." *Clinical Perspectives in Gastroenterology* 2:40-46, Jan-Feb 1999.

INDEX

A

abdominal pain, 20, 26, 58, 71, 83, 99, 100, 103, 117, 132, 143, 155, 163, 166
abduction, 119
acid reflux, 144
angiogram, 121, 144
anorexia nervosa, 68
anti-anxiety medication, 141, 142
antidepressant(s), 129, 131, 137, 138
    medication(s), 77, 134, 137, 145, 156, 167
antidiarrhea medication, 140
anxiety, 18, 21, 38–40, 48, 50, 59, 88, 89, 108, 123, 138, 180.
    See also depression/anxiety
        disorder, 34, 38–40, 115, 140–43, 146, 147, 175, 190
            treatment of, 145
assault, 37, 69, 119, 127

B

baffling illness, 16, 24
belief systems, 49, 157
bulimia, 68

C

care delivery, 186
chemical imbalance, 38, 131, 145, 181, 189
childhood stress, 23, 26, 34, 36, 40, 55, 64, 66, 76, 77, 79, 80, 85, 172, 180, 190
    consequences of, 66, 71, 73
    survivors, 67, 68, 70, 71, 82, 95, 174, 175, 190

F
food allergy/poisoning, 149

G
gastrointestinal tract, 103
Good Partner/Bad Illness syndrome, 55, 71, 83, 94, 150, 158, 191

H
healing stress illness, 28, 40
health education, 192
HIV infection, 138
homosexuals, 159
hyperventilate, 156
hyperventilation, 141, 142, 144, 190. *See also* deep breathing

I
intestinal symptoms, 188

M
medical illness, 36
mental health clinician, 181, 191. *See also* stress medicine specialists
mental health counseling, 94, 139, 145, 146, 156, 176, 181, 182
mental health counselor, 40, 41, 87, 90, 115, 142, 146, 191
mental health treatment, 175, 177, 181, 182
magnetic resonance imaging (MRI), 30
mother-daughter bond, 153
multi-factored stress illness, 58, 148
multi-factorial stresses, 37
multiple stresses, 148, 151, 152
muscle tension, 31, 141

N

nerve disease/long-standing diabetes, 105
nerve signals, 31, 32, 89, 104, 115
neurotransmitter(s), 131, 135
    imbalance, 136, 178

O

orthopedist, 119

P

paroxetine, 141, 145
pelvic congestion syndrome, 20
pelvic inflammatory disease (PID), 151
PID infection
    transmission of, 151
plastic rectal probe, 142
post-trauma symptoms, 129
post-traumatic stress, 18, 37, 41, 48, 49, 119, 120, 127, 128, 155, 172,
  175, 180, 189
post-traumatic stress/anxiety disorder, 175
post-traumatic stress disorder (PTSD), 37, 129
    symptoms of, 119, 128
post-traumatic stress/phobias, 145
psychological therapy, 181
psychosomatic disease, 19

R

recurring cough, 30
relaxation technique, 115, 129

S

self-care time, 113

V

X

ABOUT THE AUTHOR

Dr. David Clarke received his B. A. in psychology from Williams College (Phi Beta Kappa), and his medical degree from the University of Connecticut in 1979. Since then he has successfully cared for thousands of patients with stress illness, often sent to him after other doctors were unable to help them. He has been a visiting professor at several international hospitals, including Oxford. He was also named a Top Doctor in the *Portland Monthly* magazine physician review in 2005 and 2006.

Dr. Clarke is a Clinical Assistant Professor of Medicine with Oregon Health and Sciences University, a Clinical Instructor at Pacific University, and a member of the Academy of Psychosomatic Medicine. He is board-certified in Gastroenterology and Internal Medicine, and has practiced in Portland, Oregon since 1984. He is a Gastroenterologist at Kaiser Sunnyside Medical Center, he is Ethics Director at Northwest Permanente, and he is Nutrition Support Team Director at Kaiser Sunnyside Medical Center.

David Clarke has received numerous awards for excellence in patient care. He developed and presented a monthly seminar on stress illness, and local doctors have given their patients tens of thousands copies of his brochure on this topic. He lives in Happy Valley, Oregon, which is near Portland.

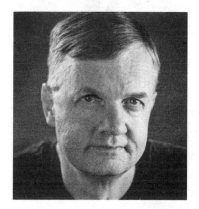

Sentient Publications, LLC publishes books on cultural creativity, experimental education, transformative spirituality, holistic health, new science, ecology, and other topics, approached from an integral viewpoint. Our authors are intensely interested in exploring the nature of life from fresh perspectives, addressing life's great questions, and fostering the full expression of the human potential. Sentient Publications' books arise from the spirit of inquiry and the richness of the inherent dialogue between writer and reader.

Our Culture Tools series is designed to give social catalyzers and cultural entrepreneurs the essential information, technology, and inspiration to forge a sustainable, creative, and compassionate world.

We are very interested in hearing from our readers. To direct suggestions or comments to us, or to be added to our mailing list, please contact:

SENTIENT PUBLICATIONS, LLC
1113 Spruce Street
Boulder, CO 80302
303-443-2188
contact@sentientpublications.com
www.sentientpublications.com